Free
Rein
to Kill

Free
Rein
to Kill

◆

Euthanasia in America

Paula Andrasko
Madeline Kisha

iUniverse, Inc.
New York Lincoln Shanghai

Free Rein to Kill
Euthanasia in America

iUniverse books may be ordered through booksellers or by contacting:

iUniverse
2021 Pine Lake Road, Suite 100
Lincoln, NE 68512
www.iuniverse.com
1-800-Authors (1-800-288-4677)

The information presented in this book is not to be construed as medical or legal advice. Suggestive tips throughout the book are only that and are used at your own risk. In the event you use any of the information in this book regarding yourself or another person, the authors and the publisher assume no responsibility for your actions.

ISBN-13: 978-0-595-34041-5 (pbk)
ISBN-13: 978-0-595-78830-9 (ebk)
ISBN-10: 0-595-34041-5 (pbk)
ISBN-10: 0-595-78830-0 (ebk)

Printed in the United States of America

DISCLAIMER

The names of the doctors and other medical professionals in this book have been changed to protect the individuals, hospitals and agencies involved in the wrongful death of our father. We have done so to protect ourselves because although we do not have the right under Florida law to sue the doctors, they could still sue us.

Hospice as used in this book is not the name of a real agency. It is used generically to represent a movement and to protect the identity of the actual agency that was involved in the treatment of our father.

◆   ◆   ◆

For our father, Paul Joseph Vertucci, Sr.
Your kind and generous spirit is giving still.
We love you!

◆   ◆   ◆

Contents

Preface xi

Introduction xiii

Part I   Liberation

CHAPTER 1   On our Way to Dying. 3

CHAPTER 2   Releasing Tears to Heaven. 7

CHAPTER 3   Symbols of Love and Unity 9

Letter: Letter from Harry S. Truman. 11

Part II   A Courageous Battle

CHAPTER 4   Responsibility 15

CHAPTER 5   A World of Vision. 18

CHAPTER 6   Tactics and Delays. 21

CHAPTER 7   A Birthday to Remember. 24

CHAPTER 8   Complications. 29

CHAPTER 9   The Power of Angels 33

CHAPTER 10   Nine Hours. 38

CHAPTER 11   Making Peace 41

CHAPTER 12   The Anointed 47

CHAPTER 13   The Road to Recovery. 52

Part III   Into the Light

CHAPTER 14   The Power of Light 57

CHAPTER 15   End Stage? 59

CHAPTER 16   "Death Warrant" 63

CHAPTER 17   Euthanasia 69

CHAPTER 18   Into the Light. 74

CHAPTER 19   The Heart of the Matter. 76

Poem: Into the Light 80

Part IV   Recompense

CHAPTER 20   The Hippocratic Oath? 87

CHAPTER 21   Disbelief. 90

CHAPTER 22   A Call for Justice 92

CHAPTER 23   Epilogue to Euthanasia. 95

Acknowledgements 101

Doctors' Acknowledgement. 103

About the Authors 105

APPENDIX. 107

Index 111

Preface

This book is dedicated to the memory of our father, Paul Joseph Vertucci, Sr., who was taken from this world prematurely.

Dear Dad:

You were winning your battle with cancer. You were in remission and ready to start another round of radiation, but a managed health care system wrote you off and signed your death warrant. You were still a stage-three cancer patient in remission when the doctors callously changed your diagnosis to end stage. They sent you home with hospice care to get you off their books.

We fought for you, Dad, and we're sorry that we couldn't stop what happened to you. You had so much more to give this world in terms of compassion and love, kindness and generosity, joy and happiness. We are sorry that the world has lost what you had to offer.

You always said it was important to give to people and be kind. You understood the true purpose of life: to love and to serve others. At your funeral, we passed out Bibles as your last gift to those who came. This was our way of allowing you to give to people one more time.

We are sad that you are gone, Dad. We will miss seeing your smiling face and hearing you sing to the birds on your back porch, but we know you are with us in spirit. We offer this book in memory of you. The medical bureaucracy that sent you home to die didn't honor you or realize your worth as we did. They saw only your outward form. They saw you as an eighty-year-old man with cancer who had used up too much money. You didn't look good on their books. They didn't know that the bottom line isn't about money; it is about love, and you were loved and are loved more than you will ever know.

Until we meet again in Heaven, know that you are still alive in the hearts of your family and the many, many others whom your life and love have touched. Even though you are gone, you are still giving to others. This book is a continuation of your love and generosity.

Your loving family,

Paula
Joe
Allan
Maddie and Kirk
Lynn

Introduction

In March of 2004, Paul Joseph Vertucci, Sr. was diagnosed with esophageal cancer caused by Barrett's disease and chronic acid reflux from GERD (gastroesophageal reflux disease). He underwent chemotherapy and radiation treatments to shrink his tumor as part of palliative treatment to relieve the pressure on his esophagus and extend his life by two to three years. His family was very hopeful. On July 1, 2004, after completing his first series of radiation treatments, he was a stage-three cancer patient in remission.

On July 5, 2004, he was admitted to the hospital for an impacted bowel. On July 9, 2004, he was released and sent home with hospice care. His bowel condition had not been treated. Because he was a cancer patient, and eighty, and had cost his health maintenance organization (HMO) a substantial amount of money; the doctors changed his diagnosis from stage-three remission to end stage, indicating that his cancer had spread throughout his body. There was no evidence to confirm this diagnosis, and all tests had come back negative.

• **Passive Euthanasia** entails withholding life sustaining medications and/or treatments to allow a person to die.

• **Involuntary Euthanasia** entails the administration of pain management and other drugs against one's will. The end result is murder.

His daughters, Maddie Kisha and Paula Andrasko, fought with the doctors regarding this misdiagnosis. They would not agree to place their father in a palliative care unit where he would have been passively and involuntarily euthanized. His daughters felt at that time that he was not dying. Yes, he had cancer, but he was beating it. The doctors at the hospital, in fact, signed his death warrant when they issued a premature order to send him to palliative care. When the family refused, they released him with in-home hospice care. His daughters were not given a third option, a home health care aide, which would not have included the death-oriented comfort care and pain management protocol of hospice.

Vertucci's daughters were also concerned because he had been over-medicated for blood pressure and pain. Based on these concerns, his medications were readjusted and he was taken off pain medicine. At home, his daughters continued to battle with the hospice nurses over this same issue. Vertucci was sent home with liquid Roxanol (morphine) and Ativan, which is contra-indicated when morphine is given. He was not experiencing cancer pain but still complained about his abdominal problem, which had been left untreated. Vertucci was doing well and improving until a double dose of morphine and Ativan worsened his condition.

On July 18, 2004, Vertucci died from drug-related complications. Morphine shuts down the kidneys, resulting in renal failure. It also shuts down the respiratory system and stops the heart. Vertucci was still in remission from his cancer when he died.

According to Floridians for Patient Protection, thirty-one Florida residents die every day from medical mistakes. That translates into 11,315 Floridians a year. Vertucci was just another victim, but without rights under the law.

The Florida Wrongful Death Act limits medical liability awards to the following groups:
- Spouse
- Minor child*
- Parents of a minor child*
- Partly or wholly dependent* blood relatives and adoptive brothers and sisters

*A minor child or dependent must be under twenty-five years of age.

The Florida Wrongful Death Act protects doctors, hospitals and HMOs from wrongful death claims. In Florida, you cannot sue for wrongful death or malpractice unless you are the spouse or a minor child under twenty-five years of age. This gives doctors, hospitals and HMOs free rein to do whatever they want. In the case of Vertucci, it meant changing his diagnosis and overdosing him. The nature of hospice care is to withhold life sustaining medications and/or treatments and to medicate the patient for comfort care only. This, in essence, is passive euthanasia. In the case of Vertucci, where drugs were administered against his will and the will of his family, it was nothing less than involuntary euthanasia or murder, and under Florida law this is allowable.

This is the story of Paul Joseph Vertucci, Sr. and his daughters, Maddie Kisha and Paula Andrasko, and their fight to get him medical attention and to keep him alive. In the end, their determination and love were not enough. An agnostic medical science and the new wave of bioethics won out. Vertucci was looked at as having no intrinsic value as a human being. He was not a spirit in a body, but just a body. This approach to medicine has usurped the medical ethics of the Hippocratic Oath. No longer are doctors practicing healing; instead they worship the bottom line mentality of a managed health care system. Modern medicine is primarily about dollars and cents and not about human worth and healing. There is a movement afoot about the right to die, but what about the right to live, regardless of one's age or state of consciousness? We face a holocaust in health care. If one man can be effectively euthanized to offset the bottom line, what then of the many baby boomers who will soon approach retirement? Will they not be too costly to keep on the books?

Vertucci's daughters have dedicated themselves to educating the American public about euthanasia and other relevant death and dying-related issues. What is going on in health care today is worthy of grave concern. This is a war, and men and women like Vertucci, who fought to keep their country free for democracy, are losing it. Join us in taking action to stop the killing.

Please check out the last chapter of this book and the Appendix for information about what you can do and for a listing of websites where you learn more about these life and death issues.

There is no doubt about it. The holocaust is coming. It is our responsibility to be awake and aware. No one else can do it for us.

PART I
Liberation

Courage is the inner fortitude that
allows men to overcome their fear and fight back
when fate demands it. Without courage there can
be no peace.—Paula Andrasko

1

On our Way to Dying

The last time we saw our father, he was in a green marble box. Maddie was holding his ashes on our way to the Florida National Cemetery in Bushnell. A World War II emblem was engraved in gold under Dad's name.

Paul Joseph Vertucci, Sr.
Born May 9, 1924
Died July 18, 2004

Maddie was wearing Dad's watch in memory of him. It was too big for her, but it still told time. Time had no meaning for us anymore. Without our father to guide and protect us, time was empty. The black hand of the watch whirled around along a preordained path. It made about as much sense as the black and white swirls that embellished the green background of Dad's urn. Within its cold, hard walls lay the last remains of the man who had been known lovingly as Pauley.

Florida National Cemetery is one of a hundred and twenty national Veterans' cemeteries in the United States. For more information about the locations of these national cemeteries visit http://www.cem.va.gov/nmc.htm. Using the sites' Nationwide Gravesite Locator, you can locate specific gravesites. You can also find helpful information about Veterans' Burial Benefits on this website.

It was a long drive to the cemetery. The limousine was full. We three daughters, Paula, Maddie and Lynn, shared our silent grief as we drove the endless miles of Florida highway on our way to Bushnell. No one spoke. Words were inadequate. Even the brilliance of the noonday sun couldn't soften the depths of our sorrow.

As we entered the cemetery, an American flag and a solitary row of bushes greeted us. This was a day we weren't prepared to meet. It was a day that should not have happened yet. We were angry and upset, sorry and depressed. This was the day we would lay to rest a great man, our father, who had fathered us and fought for our freedom. Dad had been proud to serve his country in World War II. He had fought in Germany and helped to liberate Ohrdruf.

As the honor guard paid tribute to this gentle hero, they draped the American flag he had defended so bravely over his urn. It was a moment of silent reverence for a man who had meant so much to his family. Dad was a lifetime member of the Veterans of Foreign Wars (VFW) and on many occasions had worn his VFW hat, as did the honor guard today in memory of the many veterans who had given their lives for their country. The ten members of the honor guard had never met our father, but they showered him with the respect that was due him. Even now, he was touching people's lives as he had done all his life.

There was a woman in Germany who never knew his name, but he had helped her during the war. He led her along war-torn roads as she was about to deliver her first child. Dad had found her among the collapsed buildings of a German town the Americans had just taken. When Dad took her to the medics, they chided him, "Get her out of here."

Dad was determined to get her help. He didn't see her as the enemy. She was a woman with nowhere to give birth. He somehow convinced the American medics to help this woman. He would never know her child's name or what would happen to them, but his courage and love would touch their lives for the rest of their lives.

Dad was a man of honor and integrity. Like this unnamed woman, he had touched many people during his lifetime, but today, July 18, 2004, his journey was over. In what was a brief ceremony, we said our last goodbyes. We came together in one of the isolated committal shelters where families could pay their last respects. This place, nestled among almost 513 acres of consecrated land, was designed like a tent to remind us of the tents that once sheltered servicemen like our father during the war.

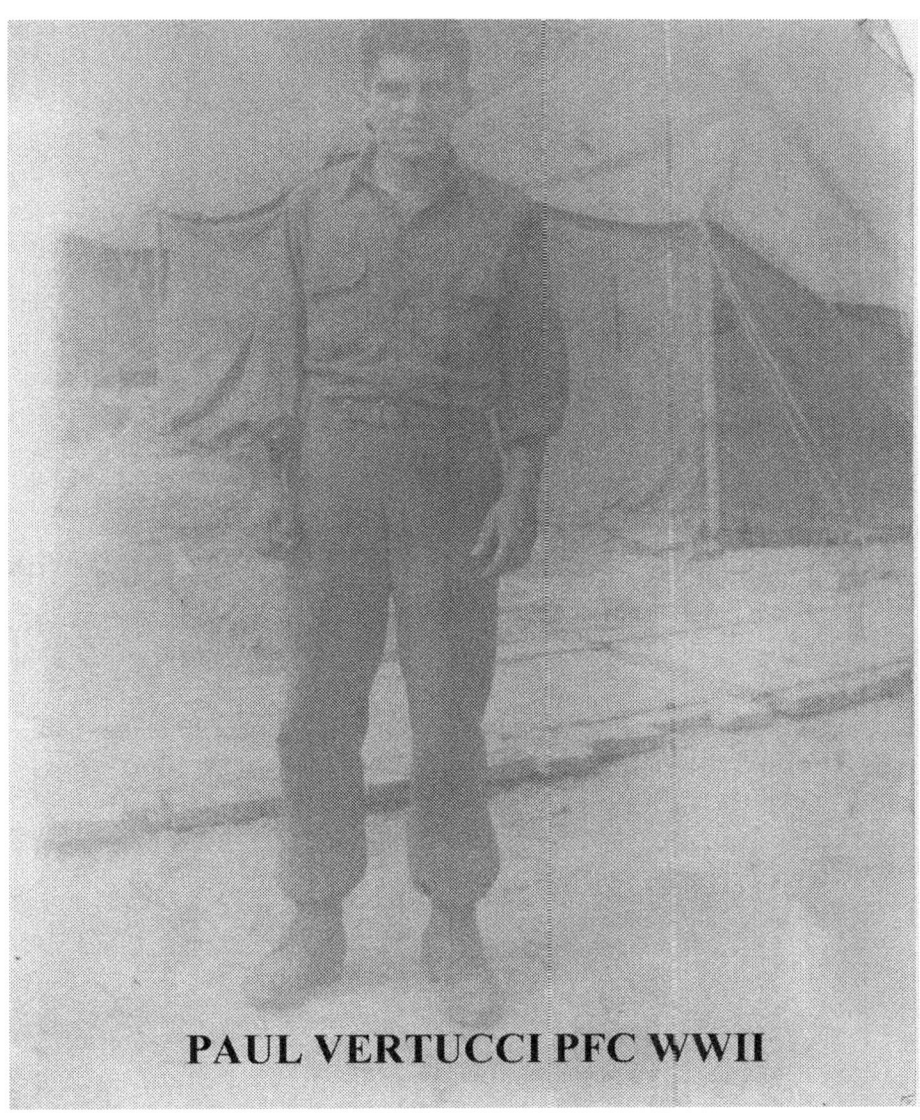

PAUL VERTUCCI PFC WWII

Dad was familiar with tents and trenches. His days during the war had been harsh. He had known about death and dying too. As a young man, barely old enough to be a soldier, he had watched as other young men like himself were being blown up all around him. He saw body parts flying through the air like debris reminiscent of September Eleventh. Bodies were being catapulted through the air, falling to the earth below where other bodies laid in agony and death. In an hour as a nation, we faced what our brave fathers and grandfathers had confronted on the road to stop Hitler.

We can only imagine our father's fear as his regiment marched toward Hitler's stronghold. As he was crossing the Rhine River, machine gun fire blazed through the brimstone air. Bodies were falling all around him, some dead and wounded, others swept away by the turbulent waters. All this blood and glory seemed like a gateway to hell. The lives of those stalwart, young men were shattered by bullets and hate, ripped apart by war and prejudice. Dad was haunted all his life by the sound of those brave soldiers crying out for their mothers as they faded into eternity.

Our father and his fellow servicemen had paid a high price for peace. Today, almost sixty years later, we were gathered together to pay tribute to him. This would be the last time we would see this man who had fathered us in the patriotism and the love of his country that was so important to him. He was dead and about to be buried, and it was still inconceivable that he could have been taken from us so callously and so soon. Dad had fought his battle with cancer courageously. He wanted to live. "I'm not ready to die," he insisted.

Dad was determined to win his battle against esophageal cancer. The odds were against him, but his determination was strong. Dad was eighty but he was a young eighty, full of life and vigor. He loved to give to people and help others. His generosity was endless, and his kindness was well-known. But his determination would be lost in the bureaucratic trenches of redtape and paperwork of a managed health care system that would cost him his life. Dad was only a number on their bottom line; but on his way to dying, this man of courage and faith, Paul Joseph Vertucci, Sr., had served both his country and his family well.

2

Releasing Tears to Heaven

After the eulogy, Maddie went to the podium to say a few words. She thanked everyone for coming and spoke of her father with words of love and tenderness. Maddie had been Dad's caregiver, and they were very close. Maddie returned to her seat, and the honor guard continued the service. The only woman in the guard ceremoniously folded Dad's military flag into the death triangle, a symbol of the unity of Father, Son and Holy Ghost.

Next, the seven honor guards who were outside the committal shelter shot off a salvo of blanks in a twenty-one-gun salute. The sound ripped the skyline like the tears that riveted their way down the faces of Pauley's family. In three identical salvos of seven shots each, the seven guards let out their brief explosion of sorrow for a man they had never known. They shot off seven simultaneous blasts, then seven more and then a final seven. The sound of Taps filled the tent and pierced our hearts like the blank rounds that had preceded it, and then it was done.

After the ceremony, the family searched with the guards as they looked for the empty cartridge casings. Altogether they found ten. Three were placed inside Dad's flag, and the other seven were given to Maddie as a token of remembrance.

Afterwards, we made our way to the gravesite. Bushnell is massive. It winds around in turns and twists where fields of crosses, hundreds and hundreds of crosses, stand out against the trees. This was a sacred place. Sixty-three thousand soldiers, veterans from almost every war, are buried here: the Spanish American War, the Civil War, World Wars I and II, Korea and the Vietnam War. The fresh grave of a soldier killed in Iraq was not out of place here among the honored dead. The harsh reality of death was disguised by the pine trees and granite markers that made up this place. It was a good place and it was a bad place.

We made our way to Section 323 where Dad would be buried. By the time we arrived, a man was already digging Dad's grave. Time seemed endless in those few minutes it took for him to remove the dirt from the gravesite.

Maddie, in a pink polka dotted black dress, stood with her family. Dad's watch hung loosely around her wrist. We were alone in our grief. Our father was dead, like our mother before him. Now Mom and Dad were both gone, and there was no one left to guide us and protect us. We had loved our parents very much. Mom preceded Dad in death by thirteen years. She suffered a long and agonizing death. Dad's suffering had been briefer. It had been ended prematurely by those who were charged with his healing.

Mom was buried in Ohio. Her ashes would remain there. In memory of her, the words "Together Again with Vi" would be placed on Dad's tombstone. Those poignant words would bind them together in death, but in our hearts and minds they were together as they had always been: in the love of Christ.

3

Symbols of Love and Unity

The words of a letter from a chaplain during World War II seemed more meaningful now. We found his letter in Dad's war picture album. It was addressed to his sweetheart Viola as his regiment was preparing to leave for active duty in Europe. The chaplain assured Viola that her sweetheart Pauley had gone to Communion and was ready for departure from Camp Miles Standish in Massachusetts. Strengthened by the grace of God, this brave young man could find peace during these times of separation and uncertainty.

On Dad's way to Germany and the atrocities of war, an army chaplain had bound our father and mother together with his generous words of hope and love. Today, they would be forever together again in a place where separation and anxiety could no longer harm them.

When the gravedigger was finished with Dad's grave, Maddie handed him Dad's urn. Dad was buried in a shallow grave. His great granddaughter Sara stood solemn watch as the dirt was shoveled over him. Her heart was broken. Earlier, when she had heard the twenty-one-gun salute, she had cried out, "They shot Great Grandpa behind the wall!" A child's sadness was loud and clear. Her pain was undeniable.

After Dad's burial, we prayed the Lord's Prayer. Then Sara and her sister Kiley walked together hand-in-hand, carrying a red balloon. We each had signed the balloon and written something on it as a final message of our love:

"Dad, you will always be with me, with all my love and heart."

"I love you."

"Kisses to heaven for Great Grandpa."

"Love you, gramps."

"You are so special to us all; we miss you (BTO) Big Time Operator!"

"Thank you for the many gifts you gave us: love and kindness, generosity and compassion, joy and creativity."

"I love you, Dad."

"You are the sweetest man; you are missed."

"You are helping Jesus now."

"We love you. We miss you. Don't leave us."

Up! Up! Up! The heart-shaped balloon rose into the sky, up toward the sun, up to the heavens, up to the place where Dad and Mom and God were one.

Paul J. Vertucci

To you who answered the call of your country and served in its Armed Forces to bring about the total defeat of the enemy, I extend the heartfelt thanks of a grateful Nation. As one of the Nation's finest, you undertook the most severe task one can be called upon to perform. Because you demonstrated the fortitude, resourcefulness and calm judgment necessary to carry out that task, we now look to you for leadership and example in further exalting our country in peace.

Harry S. Truman
The White House

PART II
A Courageous Battle

The face of courage often goes unnoticed
in the darkness of man's inhumanity to man.
—Paula Andrasko

4

Responsibility

When Paula, Joe and Maddie protested the Vietnam War in the early seventies, Dad had been angry with them. He had risked his life to free the world from Hitler. They didn't understand the horror of the Holocaust. But even though they hadn't agreed with him, they still respected him; and he never rejected them because their beliefs were different from his. Tolerance and respect are mutual ingredients of love. Dad knew that someday his children would understand what he knew about the past: Germany and Vietnam were two entirely different places.

> Visit http://www.ushnm.org/ to hear first-hand testimony from a Holocaust survivor. History is important. The past preserves the present.
> - Take time to listen to a soldier's war stories.
> - Tape his stories or write them down.
> - Create a scrapbook of her photographs and letters.

When we were little, Dad would tell us war stories. In the middle of a thunderstorm, we would dive for cover as he reminisced about his days in combat. He didn't share the gory details, but his fear and suffering spoke for itself. Dad suffered incredibly because of the horrors that he experienced. What he saw and what he witnessed left an indelible mark on his life. He would be haunted many years by the memories of all the death and torture along the road to victory.

When Dad was in Germany, he came face-to-face with the truth of man's inhumanity to man. When the Soviets were on their way to free Auschwitz, Dad's company was on its way to liberate Ohrdruf in Germany. They saw indescribable terror and things best left unspoken. Along the road to liberation were villages filled with ordinary people. They had to hear. They had to smell. They had to see.

"How could no one know?" Dad once asked Maddie as they were talking about the war.

"You could smell the stench of the dead bodies everywhere." When the Allies liberated Ohrdruf, they found bodies stacked in barracks. Others were lying on the ground, shot in the back as they were trying to escape before the Allied liberation.

Why didn't someone speak up and try to save these people? Eleven million people died by Hitler's order. Six million were Jews. Dad wasn't responsible for what these people didn't hear or smell or see, but it haunted him the rest of his life.

Dad ended the war in a building that blew up around him. He was asleep and the next thing he knew he was in the hospital, and then it was all over. The Allies had freed Germany, and Dad was a war hero. He was awarded the Bronze Star for his service to his country, but during the seventies and the Vietnam War no one seemed to care. They didn't remember the price he had paid for peace, and what kind of courage it took be a soldier. Patriotism didn't seem to matter then, but it did to Dad.

Dad was a good man who fought to free other good men from tyranny and evil. He was a hard-working, honest and diligent man. After the war, he got married and raised a family. He served as an usher at his church and did woodworking for the priests, but he never forgot what he had seen in the war. Dad suffered from post traumatic stress because of the war, but despite his own condition he was always good to people. When he was diagnosed with esophageal cancer in March of 2004 we were so sure that he would beat it. Even though his cancer was very aggressive and incurable, we prayed for healing and never lost hope. Paula wanted a miracle, and no one could take away her right to believe in one. When Paula lost her job, she came to Florida to help Maddie during Dad's chemotherapy and radiation treatments.

"No one can steal my hope," Paula insisted. "It's mine and it's immovable." No matter what anyone said, she was unshakeable.

We had a series of miracles along the way, the first of which was Paula losing her job. It happened on the day before she was scheduled to go on vacation. If it hadn't been for that seeming coincidence, she wouldn't have been able to spend the last nine weeks of her father's life with him.

Paula came to Florida armed with confidence in the healing power of God and left with a peace beyond understanding. It wasn't the world's peace. It was God's peace, and even though her miracle had been stolen from her by the bioethics of a managed health care system, they couldn't steal her faith. Dad didn't die from his cancer. He was stage-three remission when he died. His cancer had stopped growing. It hadn't spread. Dad was winning the battle as we awaited the next series of radiation treatments that would shrink his tumor. Dad once told Maddie, "If I could survive World War II, I can survive my cancer."

Dad's determination was strong, but the doctors misdiagnosed him as end-stage metastasized and assigned him to hospice care. They ignored his impacted bowel and stopped his radiation treatments. We fought for our father, but it wasn't enough. He was involuntarily euthanized in a country where euthanasia is illegal.

Was Dad's death an isolated death or medical mistake? How many others have died or will die as he did? Is there another holocaust brewing in America? Was he just the forerunner of another wave of intolerable inhumanity? When the baby boomers reach retirement, will there be too many of us for an already overburdened health care system? Will the price tag be too high and will the new wave of bioethical doctors declare us end-stage and relegate us, as they did our father, to palliative care or hospice care and send us home to die?

Can we not hear or smell or see? Who is responsible for what has been done and what is to come? Are we prepared to take action or sit back passively and wait for the slaughter? On the road to Tallahassee or Columbus or Albany, will we arm ourselves with the truth and prepare ourselves for battle or will we let uncaring people steal our hope and kill us one by one, sending us into the shadows of a false comfort care where no one will ever notice? The choice is yours. The choice is mine. The responsibility is ours.

5

A World of Vision

The eyes are the mirror of the soul. The first time Dad looked at his baby daughter Paula, he saw the beauty and the hope and the unlimited possibility in the depths of her penetrating brown eyes. The first time he held her he knew she was special. And even though he loved each one of his five children, Paula would always hold a special place in his heart because she was his first-born; but Maddie was his strength. She would be his rock and comfort during his old age, and she would be his advocate and protector during his days of dying. Paula would always hold that special place, but Maddie would hold his heart.

The first time baby Paula saw her father, she saw his big brown eyes filled with the light of love emanating from them. The last time Paula saw her father, his eyes expressed the entirety of his life in a single moment. His eyes opened wide for the first time in days, and he had sight again. In that brief moment he wasn't blind anymore, and the love of his family as they surrounded him was the most beautiful thing he had witnessed in his lifetime.

Beauty is in the eye of the beholder. When we lose one sense, our other senses become more acute. Blind people can't see the beauty all around them, but they can hear it and smell it and feel it. Sometimes by closing our eyes and looking into the silence within, we can sense the depth of beauty that surrounds us. It's this inner sense of knowing that allows us to transcend our limits and appreciate the truth of God's creation.

A few years after Dad moved to Florida, he lost most of his sight. Although he was legally blind, he didn't let it stop him from enjoying himself. Dad had always been an active person. He loved to bowl and golf and shop. Being legally blind didn't stop him from leading an active life or from appreciating the beauty in his world. He may have lost his sight, but he didn't lose his vision.

Dad's blindness was due to macular degeneration and diabetic retinopathy. He could see all around him, but the center of his vision was blurred. In February of 2002, he went to Birmingham, Alabama, for nine weeks to attend a blind school where he would learn adaptive skills.

During his time in Birmingham, Dad toured a museum with fellow members of a local Veteran's Administration (VA) group. It was a touching tour that the museum had created for blind and visually impaired persons. For the first time in his life, Dad would view the impressionistic works of Claude Monet in a new way. He felt Monet's expression and experienced his excitement in a reproduction of a seascape that sat beside the real one.

On this tour, Dad was able to pick up paintings, to touch them, to experience them in a way he'd never previously done. Without sight, he could see the paintings clearer than many of us with sight. Later, when Dad told Maddie about the tour, he said that everyone should experience art as he had. "Maybe it would make them appreciate life more."

Dad took this lesson, seeing and appreciating, and shared it with those around him. His life was a tapestry of beauty. He couldn't see the birds on the back porch where he loved to spend his mornings, but he could appreciate their beauty. One particular bird was special to him. Each day this black bird would perch on a limb and sing to Dad, sometimes whistling, other times almost talking. Dad would respond in kind. It was this very same bird that came looking for Dad after his death. Their universal bond was a connection that was eternal and ethereal. That was what Dad had seen in the tactile reproductions of the great masters: the timeless, universal connection between artist and creation, among all of God's creation.

> **Dad loved whistling to the birds. He always said, "Birds are God's messengers."**

Two years later, when Dad returned to the blind school, this time in West Palm Beach, he would take his compassionate and appreciative view of life with him in search of people to share it with. But this time, his expression of beauty and goodness would be interrupted by a most unwanted intrusion.

In March of 2004, Dad went to West Palm Beach for nine weeks of computer training. At the end of the training, he would receive a brand new computer. Dad was excited, but he didn't like being away from his daughter Maddie. Dad hadn't been feeling well. His long-time GERD had progressed to Barrett's disease and turned cancerous. During his stay in West Palm Beach, the doctors found a one-centimeter tumor in his lower esophagus near the stomach. It was located near the juncture where the aorta and the trachea are situated, which made it very serious.

Bioethics is the trend in modern medicine that views life in terms of Quality of Life as opposed to Quantity of Life. Its utilitarian approach values life not in terms of an individual's merit or intrinsic worth but based on their value to society. Cost-containment and managed healthcare are its primary concerns. It gives HMOs and insurance companies control over healthcare.

Dad's cancer, adenocarcinoma, was very aggressive and incurable, but it was treatable. The doctors at the VA wanted to start radiation and chemotherapy immediately. Dad wanted to go home. He wanted to talk to his daughter Maddie before he did anything. This delay would be costly but not insurmountable. His cancer was growing at a very fast rate. Within a month's time it would double and then more than double again. By May it would be five centimeters but still treatable. What would get in the way of Dad's prognosis, ironically, wouldn't be the cancer itself but rather a bioethical health care system that set up roadblocks to healing. The system established elaborate health care criteria for quality of life that sometimes denied life-sustaining treatment to those who wanted it.

Dad was eighty and had a variety of other health problems that made him high-risk. He had diabetes, congestive heart failure, renal insufficiency and high blood pressure, but they were all under control. On the other hand, Dad had a lot going for him. He had a strong support system, a winning attitude and unbounded hope. Dad left West Palm Beach with the same kind of appreciation of life and beauty that he had exhibited in Birmingham, and the same zest for life.

"I'm going to beat this," he told his daughter Maddie.

Neither age nor cancer nor blindness could impede his will to live. If will alone were enough, Dad would have made it, but it wasn't. The managed health care system that administered his insurance was indifferent to will. Even the will of God meant nothing to this imperious bioethical machine.

6

Tactics and Delays

What happened to Dad was unbelievable. After leaving West Palm Beach, Maddie tried to get him into the VA Hospital in Tampa for immediate attention. Maddie and Dad went to Tampa to consult with the doctors regarding his treatment plan. It was a very hopeful visit. The doctors at Tampa were confidence they could stop Dad's cancer.

Their plan was aggressive. They were going to perform surgery to put in a feeding tube to help with nourishment during radiation and chemotherapy. Once the cancer was shrunk, they would perform an esophagogastrectomy. They would remove part of the lower esophagus, the two nearby lymph nodes that were affected and the upper part of the stomach and then reconnect the esophagus to the stomach. This was a very serious operation and would be further complicated by Dad's diabetes, but the doctors were confident. Maddie was confident too. Dad's treatments were scheduled to begin the week after his eightieth birthday. He would be admitted to a nursing home in Tampa and stay there during his treatments.

If you or someone you love is diagnosed with cancer or another terminal illness:
- Research your diagnosis and its prognosis.
- Understand the survival rates, the risks of treatment and the treatment options that are available to you.
- Do not be afraid to ask for a second option.

Meanwhile, Maddie tried to get Dad's doctor in Orlando to schedule him for treatment earlier than that, but Dr. Ivan's office didn't want to give Dad referrals to a cancer specialist. Managed care is more concerned with profit margins and incentives. The doctor's office saw Dad as an eighty-year-old man with a terminal illness, and that's all they saw. They didn't see him as a person with grandchildren and great grandchildren. His sacrifices for his country didn't matter. His love and compassion, generosity and kindness were unimportant. It was how much it would cost to treat him that mattered. They couldn't understand the loving relationship he had with his daughter Maddie, or the many others whom he had adopted as children and grandchildren. It simply didn't matter. People are unimportant in a system of managed care. It is all about cost-effectiveness and cost-containment. Dad was just another item on the bottom line.

"There is no hope," Dr. Ivan told Maddie and her husband Kirk. "Chemotherapy and radiation don't work, and don't believe anyone who tells you they do."

The doctor's words were brutal. Maddie was angry. Time was at a premium, and time was running out. Every moment that they delayed was another day, another month, another year off Dad's life. What did it matter that he was eighty? He wanted to live. He had the right to live.

Maddie and Kirk had gone to the doctor's office with high hopes that day, but they were met with resistance on every front. They left dejected. This entire medical merry-go-round was confusing. The VA had just told them there was hope, and now they were told there was none. Maddie needed Dr. Ivan's buy-in. She wanted to keep Dad close to her. If he could be treated in Orlando, he could stay at home during his treatments. It would be easier on everyone.

"Dad, you're going to make it," Maddie asserted. "You have to beat this!" The thought of a world without her father was unacceptable.

When Maddie got home, she called Paula. Paula wouldn't buy into the doctor's negativity. She would cheer Maddie with her words of hope.

"Don't listen to what they say," Paula told her. Paula knew Maddie was resolute. She never gave up and wouldn't quit no matter what anyone told her. She just needed reassurance.

"Yesterday a nurse told me this is the worse kind of cancer. There is no cure," Maddie admitted. She explained that later someone else told her they knew someone who had the same kind of cancer as Dad and beat it. "I don't know who to believe," Maddie said.

"Don't' listen to them," Paula insisted. "They aren't God. Doctors are only technicians. They run tests and made guesses."

"But I don't know who to believe," Maddie responded.

"Believe me, not because of who I am but because of who God is," Paula reassured her. "Maddie, we're both miracles." She reminded Maddie that God had given them each extra time. "He gave me thirty-two extra years simply because I asked. Why can't he give Dad ten?"

Thirty-two years ago, Paula had a near death experience. She came into the presence of God, and He had asked her what she had done with her life. Her life flashed in front of her. God told her He had given her many talents, but when she saw what her life had added up to it was "nothing."

The realization that she had done nothing with her life was overwhelming. Paula prayed "The Lord's Prayer" and pleaded with God to let her live. God let her live.

"Be patient, Maddie," Paula told her. "I'm praying for Dad. In terms of eternity, what are ten more years to God?" Maddie felt better. Paula had been right about God before. Maybe she would be right again.

Maddie called Paula almost every day. Paula would always stop what she was doing and listen. "Why is it taking so long? What if they don't get it in time? What if they can't stop it?" Maddie vented.

"God is never a day too late or a day too early," Paula assured her. Paula was confident. She knew that God was a generous God and a healing God.

Paula never doubted. She never for one moment believed that Dad would die from his cancer. She had no idea what Maddie was up against. It wasn't just the cancer that Maddie was fighting. It was a health care system that denied people treatment based on their insurance, their age or their ability to pay. It was a tight-fisted system that could delay treatment long enough so that time would run out. It had become a bioethical machine that had lost much of its capacity for compassion and healing.

7

A Birthday to Remember

In January, Maddie threw a big birthday party for her husband. Dad was turning eighty in May, and he wanted a big birthday party too. Dad wouldn't let Maddie forget for a moment that he was turning eighty.

"Remember, I'm turning eighty," he kept reminding her. "What about my party?" he would ask.

Maddie saved her money. It was going to be an extravagant party with lots of people, food and presents. Maddie was going to make sure that Dad had the biggest and best birthday party he could imagine. She would reserve the clubhouse and make reservations for about forty people. Sixty would show up. Dad's sisters and brothers, his children, grandchildren and great grandchildren were all coming. Dad had lots of friends and family. His friends from Ireland held an early birthday party in April before they left for Dublin. Dad was well-loved.

Maddie kept Paula informed about what was going on. Every time they spoke, Paula's heart would sink. She wanted to be with her father. She wanted to help him through his radiation and chemotherapy treatments, but she had to work.

"Dad's going to be all right," Paula insisted.

When Maddie told Paula people were saying that Dad was eighty and had led a good life, she cringed. Their well-meaning sympathy was fatalistic. Dad wasn't dead yet. No one knew the hour or the day except for God.

Paula looked forward to Maddie's calls. Whatever she had to say, good or bad, was the most important thing in the world. Maddie was struggling with Dad's cancer all by herself. No one knew how hard it was. Maddie was the one who had to take Dad to the doctors and for his tests. She had to grind his food and make sure he had his insulin every day. She was the one who had to work, and when she got off, come home and take care of Dad. She was the one who heard him in the bathroom choking, vomiting and suffering.

"You have no idea how much I want to be with you," Paula told Maddie.

Paula really wanted to be with her father. It was a fervent desire of her heart. She longed to be there, to help in any way she could. God's hand was visibly at work. On Thursday at four o'clock on the day before she was scheduled for her vacation, her job was eliminated.

Paula was ecstatic. With excitement she called her sister. "Do you want the good news or the bad news first?" she asked. "I lost my job," Paula teased. "The good news is I can come and help you take care of Dad." Maddie was ecstatic too.

Paula arrived on Friday, the day before Dad's big birthday party. Everything was pretty much done. Every detail was orchestrated with love. Maddie wanted this to be the best birthday ever. It was going to be even better than her sixteenth birthday when her brother's band had played, and she was happier than she had ever been.

Dad was glad that Paula was there. The last thing he had said to her when she was leaving at Thanksgiving was "Stay. Don't go." Those words were almost prophetic. Paula should have realized then that something was wrong, but she hadn't; she was here now, and that's all that mattered.

On Saturday, there was a flurry of activity as Maddie made the last few arrangements for the birthday party. There were balloons to buy and cameras to place at every table. There was a cake to pick up and decorations for the clubhouse. Maddie's son Patrick was going to take pictures of everyone with Dad and then print the pictures and frame them on the spot. His girlfriend Julie was going to help. She was one of Dad's many honorary grandchildren. It was a lot of work but just another expression of a family's love for their patriarch.

> ## Happy 80th Birthday
>
> A multigenerational celebration offers a family an opportunity to pass on the family's history and strengthen bonds between generations. The very old and the very young can forge special bonds that preserve family traditions.
>
> - Videotape special occasions.
> - Take pictures of family gatherings to capture lasting memories.
> - Preserve family traditions by creating multigenerational scrapbooks.

Maddie and Paula picked up the cake. Patrick and Julie got the balloons. Everyone met at the clubhouse to help decorate. Paula put up a collage of pictures of Dad's life on the wall behind the head table. Maddie decorated the tables with love and diligence. Her granddaughter Kiley came in bearing a bouquet of gold and blue balloons.

"The eight didn't like us," she told her grandmother. "The first one broke and we had to get another one, and the second one almost blew away."

Murphy and his law were there as usual, but it didn't matter. Nothing was going to keep this day from being perfect, not even Murphy. Kiley handed off the balloons to someone else. Paula finished her collage. Patrick set up his camera and got everything ready for the picture-taking. Maddie put the final touches on the decorations.

It was a surprise party, but it wasn't a surprise. More people came than were supposed to. The gift table was piled high and spilled over onto the floor. The buffet was plentiful with roast beef, chicken marsala, rigatoni, pasta salad, baked potatoes, vegetable medley, shrimp and salad. Dad had already eaten because he didn't like to eat in public. When the cake was served he had a small piece, just enough to satisfy his sweet tooth.

The party was wonderful. Everyone had a good time. Patrick spent most of his time playing cameraman and printing pictures. Patrick mingled with the guests, taking their pictures with Dad as someone else videotaped the party.

"Say cheese," Patrick teased.

When the camera flashed, for one split second it was like being back in New York. Dad was hugging a young girl. He was dressed in his uniform, ready to leave for duty. He was barely old enough to be in combat, but he was determined to serve his country. He stood tall and brave, his arms around this child, protecting her and showering her with his love.

"Say cheesecake," Paula teased when it was her turn.

She looked at her father with love and admiration. He was her hero, Maddie's too. Paula didn't notice that Dad looked older than he had in November. The pallor in his face and the strain of his disease was showing, but Maddie and Paula weren't ready to see it yet.

Everyone was enjoying themselves. The adults were eating and talking. The children were helping Great Grandpa open his presents.

The camera flashed again and it was April 4, 1945, and Pauley was handing a prisoner a piece of candy and another one a cigarette. It was liberation day in Ohrdruf. In the face of undeniable suffering, Pauley and his fellow servicemen did what they could to soften the indescribable suffering. They offered the starving people candy and cigarettes.

The camera flashed again, and Dad was back in the present moment, opening cards and gifts. God was blessing him in a very special way this day for all the many acts of kindness that he had shown to people over the years.

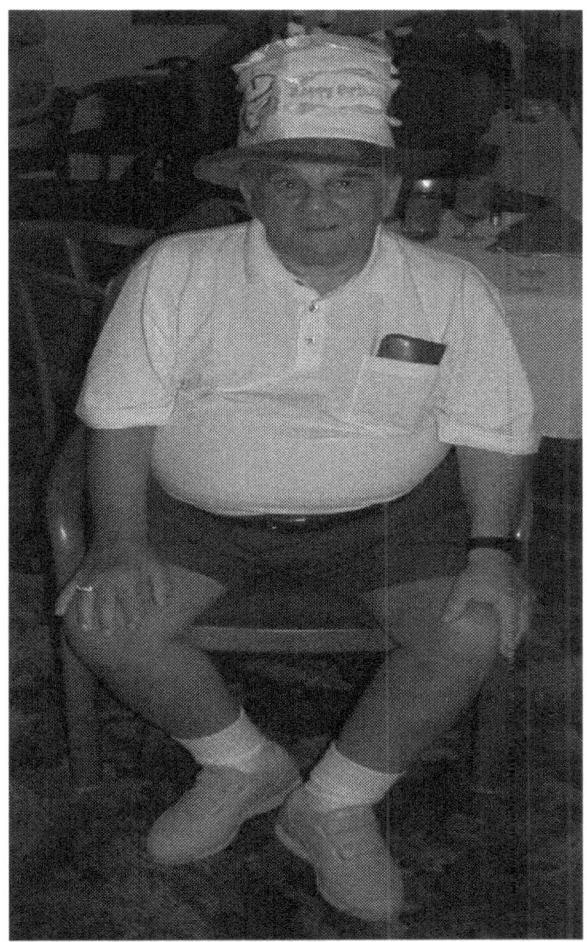

There was an endless pile of presents. Dad got shirts and shorts, expensive cologne, an "I won't grow up" beanie hat and an old man's cane with a horn. There was an electronic safe, a horn for his golf cart and a cross. There was $300 in lottery tickets and hundreds of dollars in cash. Dad was having fun despite his cancer. He wore his musical hat that looked like a birthday cake with candles that lit up. It was his crown but not his glory. His last gift was a very expensive Tiffany watch. Everyone eyed it with envy. Dad passed it around.

Today was the most special birthday anyone could have dreamed of. The anticipation hadn't been better than the arrival. The following week, Dad would be headed for Tampa to begin his radiation and chemotherapy, but for now everything was golden. Tiffany and God were both present at this special celebration for a man known lovingly as Pauley.

8

Complications

Eating was an ordeal. Dad had a five-centimeter tumor pressing on his esophagus. The opening to his esophagus was pea-sized. Maddie was the food warden. She was very careful about Dad's food. She pureed everything she could. She made bologna and egg salad sandwiches in the food processor, cutting off crusts of the bread. Everything had to be easy to swallow. Dad could choke at any time. The biggest fear with his cancer was asphyxiation.

After his birthday party, Dad's younger son Allan stayed a while. Allan liked hot dogs and pizza. He loved foot-long hot dogs with Coney sauce. One night he borrowed Maddie's truck and brought back six foot-long hot dogs. Dad really wanted one. Maddie wasn't sure. She wanted to grind his in the food processor so he wouldn't choke.

"Come on, Maddie," Dad begged.

"What's it going to do? Kill him?" Allan asked.

"Okay," Maddie agreed, "but you have to chew it really well."

Dad promised. He was so excited that he devoured the first half of the Coney dog quickly. "Can I have the rest?" he asked.

"All right," Maddie told him, "but slow down. Chew it good."

Dad wolfed the rest of the hotdog down as if it were his last meal. Shortly afterwards, he started projectile vomiting. White fluid poured from his mouth.

Paula got his spit bucket. She was scared. Maddie was scared too.

Maddie said, "I'm going to call 911."

Dad said, "No!"

Maddie called anyway. The paramedics thought Dad was having a heart attack. His blood pressure was low and his heart was irregular. He was sweating and having trouble breathing.

Dad told them, "I think I'd feel better if someone did the Heimlich maneuver." Dad had a chunk of hot dog stuck in his esophagus.

The paramedics called an ambulance, and Dad was taken to the hospital. It was Paula's job to go with him. It was an anxious ride. His blood pressure kept dropping dangerously low.

At the hospital Dad was examined, and a gastroenterologist was consulted. At two A.M., Dad was admitted to the hospital's cancer center. The eighth floor had just been opened. It was tastefully decorated and looked more like a hotel than a cancer floor.

It was a long night. By the time Dad got to his room, everyone was tired. Paula stayed, using a pull-out bed. She spent a restless night watching over her father. She wasn't sure he was going to make it. She didn't want Dad to be alone. He wasn't used to being alone. She was afraid he might choke during the night, and no one would be there to help him.

After everyone left and the lights were turned out, Dad told Paula "Good night" and said his prayers. He always prayed—almost always for everyone else, seldom for himself.

Maddie once told him, "Dad, you always pray for everyone else. It's time to pray for yourself," and they did. He wanted to get better, and he wanted his family to be happy.

Dad clutched an angel stone that Maddie had given him earlier in the week. It was a special lucky charm to keep him safe and protected. Dad had held his angel stone throughout his workup in emergency. It kept him calm. After his prayers, he put it in his pocket for the night.

The next day was a busy one with tests and doctors' visits. Meanwhile, Francis, the social worker from Dr. Ivan's office, came to see Dad. Francis was upset because no one had called their office before Dad was taken to the hospital.

Francis and Maddie were standing outside Dad's room when Paula approached. They were discussing Dad's condition. "This is a very aggressive cancer," Francis told Maddie. "It's incurable and there is no hope."

That was the wrong approach. Paula interrupted her and said, "No one is going to take away our hope."

Francis responded, "I'm only being honest."

Paula wasn't looking for Francis' kind of honesty. It was her job to be a beacon of hope. She told Francis what to do with her honesty and walked away. She went to the family room. Maddie and Francis followed her.

> ### Some Tips on Patient Advocacy
> - Discuss life and death issues before an actual crisis or life threatening illness occurs. Should you develop a terminal illness, let your family know just how much information you want to be told. This is a very personal issue and should not be decided by social workers alone. Not everyone wants to know they are dying.
> - Select someone you can trust to be your personal advocate. Choose someone who knows you well and is compassionate and sensitive to your needs and wishes. They can be instrumental in helping you throughout your illness.

Maddie was upset. Paula told her, "It's not over till it's over."

Francis sat with them. She had a point to make. This was her patient and she was in charge. "You have to tell your father he's dying," Francis told Maddie.

"We don't want to take away his hope," Maddie responded.

Francis told them, "I see this all the time. I'm a patient's advocate. Your father has the right to know."

"We are not going to tell him," Maddie asserted, "and if you do I'll sue you."

Paula told Francis, "He knows he's dying, but we don't want to come right out and say, 'Dad, you're dying.' We don't want to take away his hope."

Francis couldn't make them understand. There was no hope. She had seen too many deaths. This wasn't about hope or miracles.

For Maddie and Paula, this was about more than making decisions and handling details. This was about faith and miracles and standing on the Rock of Ages.

There are many kinds of miracles. Some happen suddenly and overtake you with their wonder. Others take time and surprise you when they happen. Still others have absolutely nothing to do with what you expect. Maddie and Paula's faith was strong. They were going to get a miracle, but it wouldn't be the miracle they wanted. The man upstairs was in charge on this one. He loved His daughters more than they could ever know, and He would ensure that they were surrounded by His love and light throughout their father's illness.

Like a small, unnamed child from a concentration camp in Terezan who wrote a poem about courage and hope, and whose life went unnoticed and forgotten by most, so too a simple carpenter from Florida—by way of Ohio and New York—would touch the lives of many, many people. It didn't matter whether or not he got a healing miracle, or whether or not he knew that he was dying. Like the child Sarah or Israel in Terezan who couldn't conceive of the possibility of dying, so too this man of fortitude and courage would leave a legacy of kindness, generosity and beauty. Christ shone in and through him, and he would enter the kingdom in the light of God; and his family would see that light as he approached it. That would be God's gift to them.

"Be good to people and be kind," Dad always said.

Even God's angels rejoiced over one so intricately and so beautifully woven.

9

The Power of Angels

What a person believes is often more powerful than what is. If one believes he is going to get well, he has a much better chance than if he believes he isn't. It's better to believe the best than the worst.

Paula believed in the power of positive thinking, but it was more than positive thinking. All the positive thinking in the world can't save anyone. It was about faith, hope and love. Paula was a survivor. Everyone in her family had at one time or another cheated death. They all had serious medical conditions or traumas and had made it through them. Over the years, Paula developed a strong and unbendable faith in God and His healing powers. It was her job during Dad's illness to affirm and reaffirm healing; and no matter what anyone said, it was Paula's duty to maintain hope.

Hope attracts positive things. That's how Doctor Gita came to us. Doctor Gita was a vibrant, positive-spirited woman with a thriving practice. She was reassuring and confident. Everyone loved her right away. Here was a doctor who was more than a car mechanic, dispensing fluid changes and new parts. Doctor Gita dispensed hope and cheer.

Upon examining Dad she told him, "I can get you to be a hundred."

Dad was elated. He told her, "Ninety."

Maddie explained Dad's situation. She told Doctor Gita that Dad was scheduled to begin radiation and chemotherapy the next week, and the doctors at the VA in Tampa were going to put in a feeding tube.

Doctor Gita said, "We can put in a stent. It will open the esophagus so your father can eat during his treatments."

Maddie was excited. She told Doctor Gita how Dad had choked on a hot dog. "We call him Hot Dog Boy," she joked.

Doctor Gita laughed. "Okay, Hot Dog Boy, we can get you to be a hundred."

"I only want to be ninety," Dad reassured her.

Everyone laughed. Doctor Gita had brought them hope.

Next, a gastroenterologist visited Dad. Doctor Bella was confident and upbeat. He scheduled Dad for the stent placement the next morning.

Paula spent the night again. When they were alone Dad asked her, "Am I dying?"

Paula answered, "No, Dad. The cancer is worse than we thought, but we're going to beat it."

Paula was upset. Dad must have heard part of what Francis had been saying earlier in the day. Pessimism is contagious. Paula stayed up with Dad until he went to sleep. It was important to keep his spirits up.

The next morning, Dad was prepped and ready for surgery. This would be a delicate situation because of the size and location of his tumor. As they wheeled him away for surgery, he was surrounded by all of his daughters. Maddie, Lynn and Paula were all hopeful that he would be all right. Maddie put Dad's angel stone in his pocket. She wanted him to think that it would be with him during surgery. After he was sedated, she removed it.

Once Dad was sleeping, his daughters went to the waiting area. They were anxious. Maddie twisted her cancer cross. It was a gold and silver cross that Dad had bought her when they found out he had cancer. She wore it every day as a sign of faith. They waited. The procedure seemed to take longer than it should. Finally, a nurse came out and said it was over.

The sisters met with Doctor Bella, who explained that he had removed a large piece of a hot dog with the bun intact from Dad's esophagus. He showed them a picture of the hot dog. "I pulled out a hot dog this size," Doctor Bella indicated by showing them the length of the hotdog graphically with his index finger. "Nothing is getting through," he told them, saying that the cancer was about five centimeters and the opening of the esophagus was pea-sized. "This is a very aggressive cancer," he said.

Before he could add, "There is no hope," Paula interrupted him saying, "Nothing can take away our hope."

Doctor Bella smiled. He told the sisters that he had tried to put a tube down their father's throat, but it wouldn't fit. Dad's tumor was large and putting so much pressure on his esophagus that the opening was very small. He told them that he was going to special-order a stent that would be big enough to open the esophagus. It would be there in a couple days, and he would bring Dad back for a second procedure.

Again, he explained Dad's chances. The rate of survival for esophageal cancer isn't good. Paula didn't care. God was working. If it hadn't been for a hot dog,

Dad would have drowned in his sleep. Getting him to the hospital because of a hot dog saved his life.

Dad was in recovery for what seemed like a long time. Once he was back in his room, he rested but he was seldom alone. Over the next several days, he had lots of company. His grandson Patrick and Patrick's girl friend Julie came with Patrick's daughters. Later, Lynn's husband and two grandchildren came. They were Lynn's step-grandchildren, but Dad was "Grandpa Paul" to them. Everyone brought gifts and laughter.

Maddie's smallest granddaughter Sara tiptoed into the room. She was afraid that she would catch what Great Grandpa had. As she entered the room, she saw Aunt Paula lying on a pull-out bed and timidly approached her. "Aunt Paula," she asked, "are you sick too?"

Aunt Paula gently reassured her, "No, Sara, I'm not sick. I'm just resting."

Sara was a little more at ease, but she was still afraid to get close to Great Grandpa. Great Grandpa let Sara's sister Kiley play with the big brown stuffed puppy dog that Maddie and Paula had bought him. They had named him "Cocoa" because he was the color of cocoa. Kiley wanted to change his name. "Let's name him Brownie," she insisted.

"No," Grandma told her, "his name is Cocoa."

When they left, Sara and Kiley wanted to take Cocoa home with them. Maddie made them leave him for Great Grandpa. Dad loved toys and all kinds of musical things. His musical teddy bear that his sister bought him was on a shelf where someone could play it for him every day. It gyrated and sang its love song when you pressed its palm. It made Dad smile.

> **Tips for Dealing with a Terminal Illness**
> - Encourage your entire family to participate in the patient's journey.
> - Allow children to be a part of the process. Be sensitive to their feelings. Reveal only as much information as the child can handle. Reassure them and don't force them to behave in ways that may be beyond their emotional readiness.
> - Rely on your faith and offer prayers and provide inspiration for loved ones. Emotional comfort care is as important as physical comfort care.

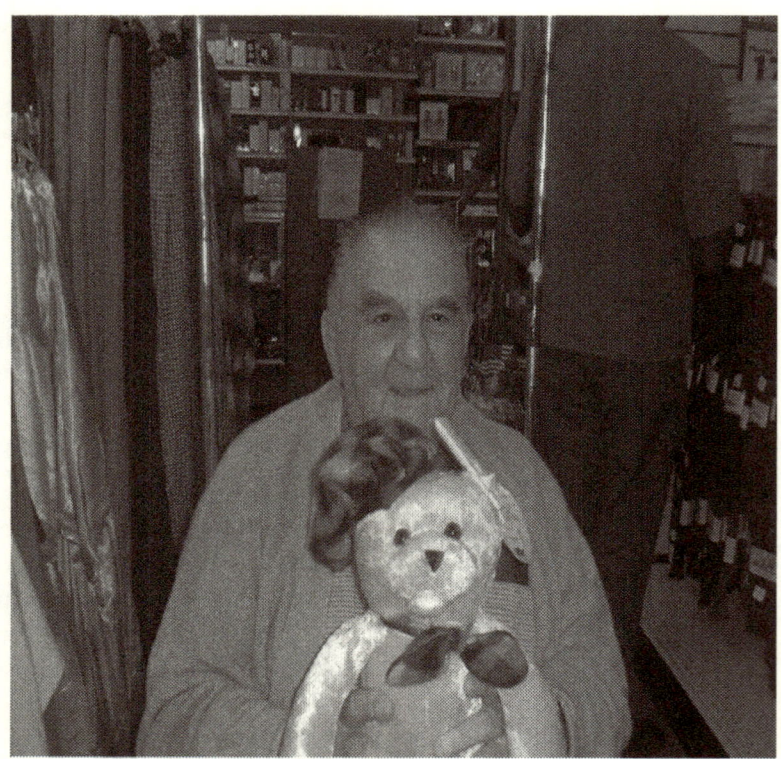

When Dad's stent came in, he was scheduled for a second procedure. This would be more serious than the first attempt. Dad would have two surgeries on the same day. The first would be to insert the stent. The second would be to put in a port for his chemotherapy and to perform a pain block. It would be a very long day, and one that would test everyone's nerves. It would be a day to call forth a flurry of angels. One tiny acrylic angel stone wasn't enough for what they were up against. This time Dad's daughters needed the power of real angels.

Paula asked Maddie if they could go to the Catholic bookstore and get Dad a statue of the Infant of Prague. She remembered the one Dad had on his night-stand when they were growing up. Over the years, it had been damaged. Lynn and Maddie had thought it was a doll and played with it. The Infant had lost his hand, and his crown had disappeared.

Paula wanted to make things right. Maddie agreed. The three sisters went to a downtown bookstore where Paula found an Infant of Prague that looked very much like the one Dad had. It had just come in that day. It was very expensive, but it was worth it. Maddie found a statue of the Archangel Raphael, the healer. Meanwhile, Lynn found a nine-hour novena to the Infant of Prague. You said it every hour on the hour for nine hours, making your request known each time. Armed with their Infant, Raphael and three novena cards, they left the bookstore.

That night, they gave Dad his Infant of Prague. They placed it on one of the shelves on the other side of his teddy bear. Raphael found a place too. If he was a healing angel, they needed him more than ever now. It wasn't that they worshipped statues. The statue was only a focusing tool. Their real faith was in God. Raphael was the archangel of healing, but Jesus was the healer.

10

Nine Hours

The first surgery began early in the morning. Dad was prepped and taken to the operating room. Maddie, Lynn and Paula waited patiently. They began their nine-hour novena, praying that Dad would "make it through the surgery."

The first surgery went longer than it should. Paula prayed that the surgery was going well. "Keep Dad safe," she prayed.

The sisters took a break outside. While they were talking, they met a woman with leukemia. She was wearing a surgical mask, which she took off to smoke a cigarette. She told them this was her second round of chemotherapy. Paula wondered why she was still smoking, but she didn't say anything.

Maddie wished the woman "luck." The woman smiled and responded, "I hope your father is going to be all right." The sisters watched her as she put on her surgical mask and went back inside the cancer center.

Novenas (Meaning Nine)

- In the Catholic faith a novena is generally a nine-day prayer for a special intention. There are novenas for specific intentions like healing.
- The novena to the Infant of Prague is an intensive nine-hour novena and is said every hour on the hour for a special intention.
- Novenas and prayers can help provide emotional and spiritual strength during times of difficulty.

Lynn looked at her watch and said, "It's time." Lynn was the timekeeper. The sisters prayed their second novena, asking God to "heal our father." The sisters finished their break and went back inside to wait.

Time went slowly. Doctor Bella was having trouble. He was having a difficult time getting the stent in. The tumor was putting too much pressure on the walls of the esophagus, but he tried again and the stent went in.

When it was over, Doctor Bella came out to speak to the family.

Lynn and Paula were on a break. He explained to Maddie that they had been successful but that it had been rough. "I couldn't get the stent down," he told her. "I didn't want to push too hard because the cancer could rupture, and then it would have been all over." He said that he had given one more try and the stent went in.

Maddie pulled out Dad's angel stone and started to put it back in his pocket. "I need to put this back before he knows it was gone," she told the doctor.

"Let me see that," Doctor Bella said. He examined the tiny angel stone and asked, "Do you believe in this?"

Maddie answered, "At this point, I'll believe in anything."

"Good," Doctor Bella responded.

Neither of them actually believed a stone could perform healing. It wasn't about lucky charms or statues. It was about faith and the strength of one's faith.

Lynn and Paula returned. They heard Doctor Bella saying, "Your father will be in recovery, and then they'll get him ready for the next surgery."

Maddie explained to Lynn and Paula what the doctor had told her. They were amazed. God was listening. It was time for another novena. They prayed for God to "heal our father's cancer."

The second surgery was scheduled at one o'clock. The sisters made their way to the main surgical waiting room. They continued their novena every hour on the hour. It helped give them a sense of control over the uncontrollable. The second surgery seemed endless. Maddie talked on her cell phone to her brother Allan, then to her other brother Joe. Lynn called her husband. The surgical receptionist told them that the surgery was over and the doctor would be coming out to talk to them. They prayed and waited. The doctor never came. Lynn checked with the surgical receptionist about Dad's condition. "He's still in recovery," he told her.

They waited. They were tired and hungry. They took another break outside. Paula noticed a blond woman across from them. She was beautiful. She had a glow about her as she sat listening to her daughter. As they were leaving, Paula walked up to the woman and told her, "Your hair is beautiful." The woman smiled. She was a lung cancer patient, and Paula's kind words were appreciated.

Maddie was on the phone again. She got thirty calls a day. It was her job to keep everyone informed. This time it was their niece Kelly from Ohio. Kelly loved Grandpa. She was his first grandchild, and she called every day to check on him.

Lynn was looking at her watch again. The sisters went back inside. They prayed their next novena. They had a couple more to go. When they were done praying, Lynn checked with the receptionist again. He told them their father was being taken to his room.

The sisters hurried to find their father. They met Dad on his way back up to his room. His bed was being pushed onto the elevator by several technicians. He didn't look good. The surgeries had been hard on him. He was still very drowsy, and he didn't know who they were.

Once settled in his room, he slept while his daughters waited and prayed. They prayed that God would "heal our father and stop his cancer."

Dad dreamed:

He was a boy again, playing handball on the streets of New York.

He was a young man dressed in his uniform waving goodbye as he headed off to war.

He was a soldier holding the hand of someone who was dying.

He was a happy groom anticipating his future.

A father holding his first child and watching her fall asleep.

A son visiting his aging father in New York.

A grieving husband crying over the grave of his beloved wife.

A father giving away his eldest daughter in marriage.

A widower moving away from his home of thirty-five years.

A loving son holding the hand of his mother as she ushered him to sleep, floating in the clouds above his bed.

As he opened his eyes for the first time after surgery, he saw a woman holding his hand. "Maddie, where is Maddie?" he asked. Maddie rubbed his hand. He was safe again in her loving care.

11

Making Peace

Their brother Joe hadn't come for Dad's eightieth birthday. He had been sick at the time. When Paula called to tell him that Dad was having an operation she reminded him, "Remember when I told you that Mom was bad, and that if you ever wanted to see her you'd better come? Well, I'm telling you that again."

"The doctors think Dad had a heart attack," Paula said.

Joe didn't say much. At the time, the doctors hadn't removed the hot dog yet. Paula explained what was going on. Something in her voice told Joe to pay attention. Paula encouraged him to come as soon as possible. Joe wanted to see his father, and even though he was still very weak, he made arrangements to fly in.

Joe flew in after Dad's surgery. Paula waited for Joe at the airport's baggage claim area while Maddie drove around. Parking was impossible. Paula watched in disbelief as a porter pushed her brother in a wheelchair. Joe looked worse than Dad.

Maddie drove from the airport directly to the hospital. Joe put on a surgical mask and went in to see his father. It had been a couple of years since they had seen each other. Their relationship had been somewhat strained over the years. The strain melted away in a minute. This was a time for healing, not just the body, but for healing relationships and making peace.

At the end of the hospital visit, Maddie, Paula and Joe went home. After the long flight Joe was tired, but he was happy to be there. This might be his last chance to spend time with his father, but he was going to make sure they did everything they could to beat Dad's cancer. "There are all kinds of new treatments," Joe insisted. If conventional medicine didn't work, they'd find something else. It wasn't about the method. It was about the results.

Dad was in the hospital eight days. During that time, Maddie decided to stay in Orlando and let Doctor Gita treat him. When she contacted the VA, they agreed. All she needed now were referrals from Doctor Ivan's office.

It was Joe's job to get the referrals. Joe had been director of a cancer institute at a medical school. Joe had the credentials to back him up. He put on his professional persona and met with Doctor Ivan. He addressed the doctor with confidence and authority. "My father wants to live," he told the doctor. Yes, he's eighty, but he's a young eighty. He wants to beat his cancer."

Maddie and Paula listened as Joe talked to Doctor Ivan, who seemed to respond to him. By the end of the visit, Doctor Ivan had given in. They had their referrals.

On the way out, Joe mentioned to Doctor Ivan that he been in the Peace Corps in Nepal. They talked about "white light." Joe explained, "People all over the world are sending white light to help heal Paul." They spoke for a while. They talked the same language. Doctor Ivan invited Joe to his meditation group the next evening. Joe thanked him.

Maddie and Paula were hopeful. Joe had single-handedly broken through the doctor's resistance. Even Jeanne from the doctor's office appeared to be cooperative. The white light was evidently working.

"Surround our servant Paul with the white light of God: healing light, soothing light, revealing light, the light of love, the light of truth. Heal our servant Paul that he might be whole and well again."

Joe stayed for three weeks. He spent most of that time recovering from his own illness. During that time, Joe and Dad made peace with each other. Dad seemed to be putting his life in order. He was gentle and apologetic for some of the things he had done in the past.

"I wish I would have been a better father," he told his children.

"You were a great father," Maddie told him. "None of us are drug addicts or in jail or homeless. You did a wonderful job."

Dad was a humble man, and even though at times his love seemed broken and imperfect, it was always real.

"You were the best father in the world," Maddie assured him.

◆   ◆   ◆

This was a very critical time for Dad. That week he began his radiation and chemotherapy. Joe, Maddie and Paula took him to his first appointment. They met with Doctor Gerald, the radiologist. Doctor Gerald was a very warm and caring physician. He explained Dad's treatment plan. He told them, "With radiation and chemotherapy, I can give your father quality of life. If everything goes well, he can live another two to three years."

Maddie was relieved. She wasn't going to lose Dad yet. That was all she wanted—just more time. Maddie knew this was a very aggressive cancer and that it was incurable, but it was treatable. Maddie wanted to believe in Paula's miracle, but if they didn't get a miracle, two or three more years was perfectly fine.

Doctor Gerald spoke enthusiastically, "I treated a patient with the same kind of cancer as your father, and he is still alive after five years."

Paula smiled. It was possible. People did make it. Doctor Gita had said she could get Dad to be a hundred. Now, Doctor Gerald was agreeing that there was hope. His optimism left them feeling better about Dad's prognosis.

On his initial visit, Dad was assessed and a treatment plan was set up. On the next visit he would be marked, and then the following day his radiation would begin. Dad would have radiation five days a week and chemotherapy every Friday.

Things looked hopeful for the first time in a long time. Maddie was beginning to buy into Paula's hope. Lynn, on the other hand, had always believed what Paula was saying because she had beaten cancer herself. Maddie had been her beacon of light. She had been with her every step of the way. When Lynn wanted to give up, Maddie made her keep going. Dad bought Maddie a cancer cross, and she wore it every day while they were battling Lynn's cancer. Lynn had surgery twice, and even when she lost hope and wanted to call it quits, Maddie was there and so was God. Maddie and Lynn knew what they were in for, but if God could heal Lynn, He could heal Dad too.

Lynn had shared her story with her sisters. "I was crying myself to sleep one night after my second cancer surgery. I kept praying, 'Lord why me? Why this kind of cancer?'

"I was so upset I told God there would be no more surgery for me. I was giving up. The pain from the surgery was horrible. That night after I finally fell asleep, I woke up in the middle of the night with the most incredible feeling I have ever felt in my life. I was reaching up and I knew that my cancer was gone.

"I went back to my cancer doctor, and he agreed that my cancer was gone and that the Lord had healed it."

Lynn knew that God had healed her. Paula and Maddie knew it too. They were all strong women. This was a very spiritual family, but not all of them were religious. Religious people can be stiff and full of unholy hearts and minds. They can be so busy singing praises and then spreading gossip after the service that they forget what the minister just said. Some of them are so worried about who's going to church and who's not, that they fail to comprehend the Gospel. Others are so full of judgment and self-righteousness, that they have very little room for love, joy, peace and patience.

Paula knew the value of worship, but she didn't like what she saw going on in the church lately. What would Jesus think if He visited them on Sunday? But it wasn't others that upset her most. Paula was angry with herself for her own unrighteousness. If she couldn't stop overeating, how could she bring honor and glory to God's name? Worship wasn't just about fifty-two hours a year. It was about the rest of the eight thousand seven hundred and eight hours when you weren't in church.

Paula was tired of the Pharisaical-minded mentality that was too busy with its own complacency and religiosity to recognize Christ in the face of a dying man. Jesus didn't come to bring religion. He came to bring salvation. God is a living God, not just a Catholic or an Episcopal or a Baptist God. God is alive and active. Paula could see how God was working, and it didn't matter what the outcome was or what others thought. She saw the signs. They couldn't.

The church was asleep. That's what the religious people in Germany had done while Hitler was taking over. They had fallen asleep and forgotten that the spirit of Christ was more important than brick and mortar. They didn't hear. They didn't smell. They didn't see. And eleven million people died.

Paula worshipped her Heavenly Father every moment. She worshipped God when she was sitting on the back porch with her Dad, when she was cleaning his room or washing out his spit bucket. God was there. She could hear and smell and see her father's suffering, and God's will for her was to be there with him and bring him a hope that was not only enduring—not just for a day once a week for a year or two—but eternal.

Paula's God, the one who had given her back her life and healed her sister Lynn of cancer, was both concrete and intangible. He was both a miracle worker and a mystery, and right now they were in the middle of either a miracle or a mystery.

Dad's family loved their father, and they wanted him to live. Life without him would be unbearable. They were looking for answers. They weren't doubting God. Some of them just wanted tangible evidence from God about Dad's chances, and God could handle that.

Lynn prayed a fleece that she would get roses in any form if Dad was going to be all right. The next day she got roses all day long. Everywhere she looked, she saw roses of joy, roses of hope, roses of healing.

The following day, Maddie prayed a prayer to St. Therese of the Little Flower. "If Dad is going to get well, send me white roses in any form." The next day, the roses would come in lots of forms and colors except white. White is for purity, and the roses she received were all pure.

On their way to radiation that day, Maddie explained to Paula what had happened to her at work. "When I left work I was feeling pretty depressed," Maddie began. "And then I looked up, and right above the building where I work was a huge sign in the sky. You know, the kind planes make in the sky for advertisements, and it said 'God.'" The plane had written 'G-O-D' in big white letters in the sky.

"See," Paula said, "God is trying to tell you something."

"Maybe," Maddie responded.

"What are the odds?" Paula asked. Sometimes coincidence wasn't coincidence. God could be very tangible.

Maddie handed Paula an envelope while they were driving. Paula opened it. "You're not going to believe this," she exclaimed.

"What is it?" Maddie asked.

It's a novena rose prayer from St. Therese, and there are roses everywhere," Paula said. Inside the prayer card there was a medallion. Paula handed it to Maddie, who put it on. Paula prayed the simple novena.

After radiation when they got home that day, Maddie's granddaughter Kiley gave her a cheer-up card. Kiley told her, "I made this just for you because of Great Grandpa." It was a hand-made card full of bright and happy things. And there were roses, lovely roses filling up its pages. Madeline handed the card to Paula.

The phone rang. It was Allan. He was coming in next week. Reinforcements were on the way. Allan would be there during Joe's last week in Orlando. It would be a time for reunions and more healing.

Tips on Grief and Grieving

Grief is an individual experience and can occur even while your loved one is still alive. The Grieving Process is a healing process and can be both sorrowful and joyous. Grief is an emotionally charged time during which you may experience a variety of feelings and emotions like anger or depression.

• Share your grief with others.
• Seek professional help for prolonged or unresolved grief.
• Be sensitive to a child's grief. Allow them to express their grief and share it in their own unique way.

While Lynn was on vacation in Ohio, the rest of them—Joe and Allan, Maddie and Paula—enjoyed a very special moment with their father. It was a once-in-a-lifetime opportunity that they would never forget. Dad was sitting on the back porch, singing to the birds. Everyone came outside to spend some time with him. They were all standing by Dad's rocker when Maddie said, "Group hug."

They weren't usually a very demonstrative family. Dad didn't always show his feelings, but Maddie's frivolity broke the ice. Allan said "Wait for the camera," and then they formed a circle and hugged. It was like being in church when they were little, with Dad carrying Allan on his shoulders while he went down to the altar for communion. It was a worshipful moment of love and healing, and the great God of the Universe was hugging them hug Dad.

During the rest of Joe's visit, he and Dad grew close. When Joe was leaving, he told Maddie, "Dad never told me he loved me so much as he did while I was here."

In the face of an incurable disease, there was time to make peace. In the arms of their gentle father, there was love and hope and faith again. And whether they got a miracle or a mystery, it would be a miracle either way.

12

The Anointed

Once Dad's chemotherapy and radiation treatments were under way, Maddie called the priest to give Dad last rites. Even though she thought he was going to make it, she wanted to make sure everything was in order.

Father King came to the house and spent an unforgettable hour with Dad. Dad showed him his room, and they talked about the war. He showed him his Bronze Star in the display case on the wall in the hallway. He was proud to have served during World War II, yet he was sad for his friends who had died crossing the Rhine River.

Dad talked about his life, about his roots in New York and his life in Ohio. He told Father King about his move to Florida and his daughter Maddie and how she took care of him. He talked about liking to go shopping and buying gifts for everyone. This was a righteous man. The father could see it in the evidence of how he lived: the love of his family, his relationship with God and his service to his country.

Father King gave Dad the sacrament of last rites. Dad was ready now to meet his Lord and Maker. He was prepared. He had been baptized, made his first communion and confirmation, been born again and received last rites. There was no doubt about where he was going.

Last Rites
• The last rites, known in the Catholic Church as extreme unction, is one of the seven sacraments. Protestants also participate in two of the seven sacraments: baptism and communion.
• Last Rites are given to the seriously ill or those near death to bring them strength, comfort, healing and repentance.

Maddie once told him, "Yes, Dad, you're going to Heaven. God has an express elevator waiting for you." She just wanted God to hold off a while.

As Father King was leaving, he told Maddie "If there's anything you need, you can call me at any time."

Maddie thanked the priest for coming. The morning had gone quickly, and it was time now to get ready for Dad's radiation that afternoon.

Monday, Tuesday, Thursday, Friday, most days were the same. Maddie usually worked until eleven A.M. and got home about eleven-thirty. She was off on Wednesday. Paula took the morning shift. She got Dad up, cleaned his room and bathroom, made his breakfast and tried to give him his medications. Some days were good and some days weren't. Some days Dad didn't want to eat or take his pills. Since he was a diabetic, it was important to control his blood sugar. If his glucose dropped below 150, Paula wasn't supposed to give him any insulin. Dad's blood pressure was also an issue. Since he began his treatments it had been dropping, and his medications had to be adjusted. His blood pressure and glucose had to be monitored carefully, but Dad wasn't always cooperative.

On good days Dad would get up early, eat and get dressed. On other days, he would sleep until ten-thirty or get up early and go straight to the back porch and then back to bed without eating breakfast or taking his pills. Sometimes when Maddie got home nothing had been done, and she would have to race around to get Dad ready for radiation. Other days Dad would say, "I don't want to go today."

Maddie remembered the time she found Dad on the back porch in his pajamas when he was supposed to be ready for radiation. Paula had tried to get him ready, but he just didn't want to go. His breakfast sat untouched on the table beside him. Eating was the hard part. You had to fight it going down, and fight it coming back up. Dad told them, "I was praying that I might eat at Jesus' table because His food would taste so good."

Maddie and Paula felt disheartened, but they got ready anyway. The treatments were exhausting. A few times they had to let Dad stay home because he was really sick or just too weak, but they were unfailing in their love and devotion. Maddie and Paula went to radiation and chemotherapy faithfully with Dad. It was tiring, but it was a labor of love. It didn't matter where or how they spent their time with him. It was time, nonetheless, and they cherished it.

Dad had radiation every day and then chemotherapy afterwards on Fridays. The big blue recliners in the chemotherapy room were comfortable. Maddie would make sure Dad had a blanket and a pillow. The nurse would flush his port and insert his IVs. He had multiple IVs. There were his chemotherapy drugs in one and Benadryl in another in case he had an allergic reaction. Another contained fluids if he got dehydrated.

Chemotherapy wasn't easy. There are a lot of side effects, and the drugs themselves are killers. They kill the good cells along with the bad cells. All the patients complained about the same things. They were always tired and nauseated. They lost their appetites. Food didn't taste good anymore. Then there was the hair loss. Some of them shaved their heads, while others wore wigs or scarves.

When Dad's hair began to fall out, Maddie took him for a buzz cut. It looked good, but he didn't like it. He kept asking, "When is my hair going to grow back?" No one could answer him. Not knowing was difficult, but Dad made light of it.

One day while Maddie was waiting for Dad she was paged to come to the chemotherapy room. She hurried back to find out what had happened. When she entered the room, there was Dad in a long, curly wig. She burst out into laughter. He stood there looking like a big gorilla in a blond wig. One of the nurses took Dad's picture and hung it up for everyone to see.

Another time, Dad played a practical joke on Doctor Gita. Lynn had found him a hot dog hat while she was on vacation in Ohio. It looked hilarious. When Doctor Gita entered the room Dad told her, "Turn around."

Doctor Gita looked puzzled but turned around. Dad put on the hot dog hat and everyone exploded with laugher.

Dad loved Doctor Gita. She made him promise, "When I get you well, you're going to take me to Coney Island and get me a hot dog."

Dad said, "I'll even pay for it."

Everyone loved Dad. His sense of humor and giving nature took some of the pain out of even the most intolerable situations. He had a heart of gold. He was a giving man and showed his generosity in all kinds of ways: like giving candy and cigarettes to a prisoner on liberation day during World War II, or giving a mother money to buy a makeup case for her little girl when she couldn't afford it, or purchasing twenty dresses and earrings at Christmas time for a battered women's shelter.

Kindness is immeasurable, but it has a tangible effect on both the giver and the receiver. Dad's random acts of kindness helped everyone feel better. He bought candy and peanuts for the nurses and patients. He made sure the candy jar was filled. His thoughtfulness emanated for the soul of a man who had seen unspeakable horror and injustice during his lifetime, but he stood up to that injustice with courage and dignity. He stood up to the hatred and indifference of a sleeping world with love and kindness.

Watching Dad undergo radiation and chemotherapy was very special. He was a "winner." At one point Maddie told him, "If it ever gets too hard and you want to quit, you can."

Dad told her, "No, then I'd be a quitter and I'm no quitter. I'm a winner."

Dad's attitude was inspirational, but his recovery wasn't always without set-backs. After only two chemotherapy treatments, his red blood count dropped. He was given weekly shots of Procrit to increase it, but he never got built up enough to have another treatment. The radiation, on the other hand, went smoothly. The cancer was being bombarded every day.

Every day the three of them, Maddie, Dad and Paula, made their solemn jour-ney to radiation. Dad would sit up front with Maddie. Maddie would blast her Christian music, and they would listen to Dad's favorite song, "Who Am I," sung by Casting Crowns. As the music played, Dad and Maddie would hold hands and Paula would cry in the back seat. Maddie wore her sunglasses so Dad wouldn't notice her tears.

Every day they drove the winding roads downtown. Sometimes Lynn would meet them at the treatment center. The waiting room was usually full. Some were patients waiting for radiation and chemotherapy. Others were there only to get their Procrit. Some patients walked in as if there was nothing wrong with them. Others had to be wheeled in, and some came by ambulance from the hospital. All had their own story to tell and their own suffering to bear.

Waiting with them, watching them endure their pain, talking to them made one so much more aware of what these patients were up against. They had every kind of cancer: colon, breast, brain, esophageal, stomach, uterine, pancreatic, bladder and lung. Sometimes it was localized, and other times it had spread. Sometimes there was hope, and other times there was only a tiny thread of hope; but even that was enough to keep them going.

As you watched them fight their battles, you became much more aware of the sanctity of life. Yes they were dying, but for today they were still alive. Wasn't each moment precious? Wasn't it wonderful to have another chance to experi-ence another day? These were the truly anointed ones, the holy ones who were near enough to touch the face of God as they underwent their daily routines and treatments.

Paula liked to sit with Dad during his chemotherapy or IV fluids. The hours were fleeting. She fell in love with the patients. The pretty blond woman who always wore the bright, perfectly coordinated outfits that were too big for her was elegant, and the room seemed to light up when she entered it. Sometimes in the silent moments, between the chatter, Paula would say a secret prayer for her.

As you sat there, it was hard not to notice the pain, the fear, the sadness of these people. They were young and they were old. They were Catholic and Bap-tist, well-to-do and poor. As Dad slept in his comfortable chair, Paula loved to share her hope with anyone who would listen. She especially liked the bald youth who had so much depth and wisdom for a boy his age.

"Never give up," she told him.

Paula told him about a child from Terezan who wrote a poem that had helped her through her own illness. "I used to walk the streets and say to myself, I won't die! I won't die! I won't die!"

An unknown child who had faced unbelievable terror had helped her through her days of dying. Before she was born, this child Sarah or Israel had written about hope under circumstances where hope was impossible. This child's courage and faith became a tangible thread of hope that helped Paula fight back.

"Pray and never give up," Paula told the eighteen-year-old cancer patient.

"It's all attitude and prayer," he said.

An eighteen-year-old boy or an eighty-year-old man, both had seen more pain and suffering in those weeks of treatment than most of us in our entire lifetimes.

13

The Road to Recovery

Dad's treatments were going very well. He particularly liked the weekends because he could stay home or go shopping. Sometimes, his two great granddaughters would spend Saturday night. Dad enjoyed spend-

> "Blow bubbles when you're sad. It makes the sadness not so bad."—Dad.

ing time with them, blowing bubbles and flying paper airplanes. He enjoyed buying them presents and spoiling them. It was fun to give them twenty dollars and take them shopping. Kiley would pick something out and then find something else and change her mind again. Sara was pretty easy. She would pick one or two things and make a choice between them. Kiley would still be moving around the store looking for the best buy. These little excursions were always fun, and Great Grandpa loved them. They gave him something to look forward to and made his treatments more tolerable.

But though Dad seemed to be getting better, he had setbacks along the way. By this time the nurses were telling us to let him eat whatever he wanted. His appetite was poor. He wasn't getting enough bulk or fluids. He was constantly dehydrated or constipated. Dad didn't seem to be in much pain. Most of his pain came from his constipation. Once in a while he would ask for Ibuprofen.

By June, Dad was having serious constipation problems. Doctor Ivan prescribed a stool softener and indicated that Dad should eat high-fiber foods and get plenty of fluids. Cancer patients have trouble eating, but it was even harder for Dad because of the nature of his cancer.

The stool softener didn't help much. Maddie gave Dad an Ex-Lax and then tried an enema. It didn't work. Later, when Dad went to the bathroom, he started coughing up blood. Maddie got frightened and called 911. The paramedics examined Dad and decided to call an ambulance. Dad was taken to the hospital. His blood pressure was extremely low again, and he was put on a heart monitor. Doctor Bella was called as well as Doctor Gita.

Maddie's husband Kirk and Paula stayed with Dad in emergency until he was admitted. The next day, Dad's social worker, Francis, came in to check on him. Francis yelled at Maddie in front of Dad, saying, "Everything has to go through our office first." She told Maddie to call Doctor Ivan's office, not Dad's cancer doctors.

Maddie was irritated with Francis. "You were not the first person I thought of calling," she told her. "My main concern was my father's health."

Paula added, "I asked the hospital to call your office." Francis ignored her and left.

Later, Doctor Bella came in. He said, "The stent doesn't seem to have moved." He indicated that he didn't want to do a scope until closer to the mid-point of radiation, and then he would re-evaluate things.

Dad was released the next day. The bleeding was because of his treatments and was normal with radiation.

After Dad's second hospitalization, Doctor Ivan's office called almost weekly to check on his condition. "How is he doing?" It seemed as if they were fishing for a reason to stop the cancer referrals. Maddie and Paula were always upbeat and positive.

Dad continued his radiation treatments. Maddie and Paula drove him there every day. They held hands and sang. They listened to "Who Am I" and cried. They talked to the other cancer patients and tried to cheer them up.

Sometimes, they would stop after radiation to pick up Kiley and Sara at summer camp. Dad would bring bags of lollipops for the teachers to pass out as treats. Everyone called him "the lollipop man." Afterwards, they would go to lunch. The girls looked forward to their special treats with Great Grandpa.

On Thursday or Friday every week, Maddie would stop for fish at Dad's favorite seafood restaurant. It was the best in town. Dad loved fish and fish sandwiches. If Dad were feeling well; they would go shopping, once or twice a week, then once a week, then every other week.

The chemotherapy was hard on Dad. His blood count continued to be low. He was on a weekly shot of Procrit and had to have a platelet transfusion. It took all morning for the blood bank to find a matching donor. While they waited, Maddie and Paula took a break in the picnic area across the street. A nurse from the hospital came up and sat with them. There were lots of empty tables, but she chose theirs. Maddie told her they were waiting while their father got a platelet transfusion. "My Dad has esophageal cancer," Maddie explained.

The nurse responded, "I have a friend who's a lawyer. He has the very same kind of cancer." She indicated that after nine weeks of radiation and chemotherapy, her friend's cancer went away. "Although it didn't cure him," she added, "it bought him some time." Maddie was encouraged.

When the nurse left, Paula asked, "What were the odds of that nurse at exactly this time sitting down at our table?" Maddie got the connection. Maybe God wanted them to know that Dad had a chance.

The rest of the day went smoothly. While Dad was having his transfusion, Maddie and Paula walked over to the blood bank across the street and signed him up. Maddie had people at work who were willing to donate blood and platelets for him.

Along with the platelet transfusion, Dad was given more fluids. He was dehydrated again. Several times in the past few weeks, he had IVs. He wasn't drinking enough, and the sun on the back porch wasn't helping.

At one point, Dad's white count became a serious issue. He had to be given Neupogen in addition to his Procrit. There was concern of infection, and Dad's immune system was compromised; but this was not unusual for cancer patients. These were all normal setbacks on the road to recovery.

At Dad's mid-way check up on July 1, he had a CAT Scan to assess his progress. Doctor Gerald asked Maddie and Paula to come back with him after Dad's radiation treatment. He said Dad's CAT Scan was good. "We put a hammer to the cancer," Doctor Gerald told them. "There is no new growth." The cancer wasn't spreading.

At that point, Dad was a stage-three cancer patient in remission. The following week, Dad was supposed to begin a second, more aggressive series of radiation treatments to shrink the cancer more.

Things looked very promising. Everyone was excited. To celebrate they stopped for ice cream. The ice cream tasted good and soothed Dad's throat. Dad was looking forward to a four-day weekend. On the way home, he wanted to go shopping. He wanted to buy Sara and Kiley toy puppy dogs that were on sale. He carefully picked out one for each of them and bought one for himself. The dogs wagged their tails and moved their ears. They were adorable.

On Tuesday after the holiday Dad would start his second round of radiation, and in four weeks he would be done. In a hopeless world, Maddie and Paula had found hope—the kind of hope that activates the kind of faith that moves mountains.

PART III
Into the Light

You have heard the angels singing.
You have touched the sky.
You are free beyond the limits of your imagination.
You have kissed the face of God and found healing
in His wings.—Paula Andrasko

14

The Power of Light

The Fourth of July is a holiday of light and independence. There are picnics, parades and fireworks. Light brightens the sky with a patriotic display of colors. White and yellow showers of light cascade down the sky. Purple and green clusters of light awaken your senses. The red, white and blue of Independence Day shouts its message of freedom and liberty.

Light is energy. It can transform one with its glory and brighten one's spirit with its boldness. Dad was full of light. Light is transforming. He could change a frown into a smile with one of his random acts of kindness like giving a teddy bear to a sick child he'd never met before. He liked to give gifts of jewelry. He gave an amethyst ring to a woman who was recently widowed, and a necklace, earrings and matching ring to his cancer doctor. He could turn a sour mood into sunshine with his teddy-bear-good-looks and melt the heart of others with his generosity and goodness. When God was handing out the fruits of the spirit—goodness and kindness—Dad purchased an orchard.

On Sunday, Maddie had a Fourth of July celebration at her house for family and friends. Her husband Kirk grilled chicken and steaks. There would be no hot dogs. Julie and Patrick and the girls brought food. Lynn brought more. Maddie's neighbor Carol brought dessert.

It was a festive day. Everyone enjoyed it. Dad was very tired that day. He slept while everyone ate and chatted. When he finally woke up, Dad was really hungry. He asked for a salad. Maddie made one, cutting everything in very small pieces. He ate the entire salad and wanted more. After supper, everyone went outside for the fireworks portion of the evening.

It was threatening to rain, and incredible bolts of lightening illuminated the darkening sky. They were like a fireworks show from God. You could feel their energy and passion.

Kirk was in a hurry to pass out sparklers before it rained. Everyone was having fun. Kiley ran around showing off her sparklers. Sara was afraid to hold the sparklers, so Kirk made it her job to pick up the burnt out ones and put them in the trash. Kiley danced around with sparklers in both hands. Sara had a fantastic time throwing them away.

Dad and Maddie sat on the glider on the front porch. Maddie lit a sparkler and handed it to Dad. Paula and Maddie watched as he twirled his sparkler in honor of Independence Day. It made them cry. Paula looked away, and Maddie turned her head. This would be the last time Dad would sit with them on the front porch. The sparkle in Dad's eyes was diminished by something that he wasn't ready to tell them. He didn't feel good and his stomach hurt, but he didn't want to spoil the celebration. He rubbed his belly. The lights of Independence Day swirled all around him. For an instant, you could almost see it. His spiritual body was shining through the tired skin of his outer form. You could almost feel its light as it connected with the moment.

15

End Stage?

After celebrating the Fourth of July with his family, Dad's condition was about to change. Dad began complaining of abdominal pain. While he was straining on the toilet, he called for Maddie.

Paula went in to see what was wrong. Dad said he wanted to go back to bed. Paula called for Maddie and Kirk. They both came running. As they tried to help him up, he started vomiting and then he passed out. His eyes rolled back in his head. He looked dazed. Kirk was afraid he was going into diabetic shock.

Paula and Maddie were frantic. They raced around like crazed people. Kirk asked for help. Paula brought a pillow to put under Dad's head. Maddie called 911.

Dad had an impacted bowel, and as a result of straining had fainted. The paramedics who examined him thought his vagus nerve had caused him to lose consciousness.

When the ambulance got there, they had a hard time getting Dad on the stretcher. They had to take him out through the back porch. Paula went with him to the hospital. As she was waiting to get in the ambulance, the attendant told her, "You can get in the truck, but we need to work on your father for a while."

Paula was shaken up. What was taking so long? The ambulance rocked from side to side as they worked on Dad. Maddie was busy gathering everything together to meet them at the hospital. It was her job to bring his paperwork, his medication list, his living will and his do-not-resuscitate order.

Maddie and Dad had talked about what he wanted if he should ever get to the point where something happened and he wasn't himself anymore. Dad told her that he wouldn't want to live like that. Maddie said she understood.

Maddie had been given Dad's power of attorney. She had taken care of all the legal paperwork. She thought she was prepared and had done what was necessary.

She didn't know that a living will could be used against you to violate your will. To the hospital, it could be an admission of your desire to end your life.

The last thing Dad said before going to the hospital was, "Could someone give me an enema?" No one heard him. Dad was taken to the hospital where he was admitted for a twenty-three-hour evaluation. He kept complaining about his stomach.

Dad was moved from emergency to the critical decision unit (CDU). His cancer specialist, Doctor Gita, wasn't consulted. In the midst of all the commotion, Maddie didn't realize that Doctor Gita hadn't been called. Dad was seen by Doctor Robert and Doctor Newman. An infectious disease specialist was also consulted. Dad had spiked a fever with an infection; his creatinine was elevated, and he continued to complain of abdominal pain.

Upon his admission to the CDU, Maddie called Doctor Ivan's office to inform them that she didn't want Francis to go into Dad's room. They could talk outside, but she was not to enter Dad's room. Maddie had enough of Francis's patient advocacy routine. She was more concerned about keeping her father alive and getting him better than dropping the bombshell: "Oh, by the way, you're dying."

During Dad's evaluation, Maddie and Paula were increasingly concerned about his medications. Paula had been saying for the past couple weeks that he was overmedicated. His blood pressure had been running low. He was on three blood pressure medicines, and the Clonidine couldn't be stopped without the risk of a stroke. At one point his blood pressure became critically low, and they were advised to monitor it every day before they gave him his medications. Maddie and Paula both insisted that his blood pressure medications be re-evaluated.

They also felt very strongly that he was overmedicated for pain. At home, he rarely if ever took his morphine. Occasionally, he would ask for Ibuprofen, and only on two or three occasions did he take a half dose of morphine. He didn't like the morphine or the way it made him feel. He also never liked the Lortab (Vicodin) that had been prescribed for him during his first hospitalization. He never took it, and here he was again being placed on Lortab and morphine. He wasn't complaining of cancer pain. He was complaining of abdominal pain. Dad was given an antibiotic for his infection; his Lasix was readjusted because of his creatinine; and his blood pressure medications were re-evaluated and changed.

One of the nurses told Paula "Your father was overmedicated for his blood pressure."

They had finally gotten the message, but they still needed to address the painkillers. Paula told Dad's nurse, "He wasn't on this much pain medicine at home.

He doesn't need it." The morphine was making him confused. He was seeing things and talking out of his head.

Maddie pitched a fit and made them take him off the pain pills. "He doesn't need pain medication," she told the nurses. "Unless he asks for it, don't give it to him."

The infectious disease specialist told Paula that her father's consciousness was impaired. Paula begged the doctors, "Wait another day. Give him one more day." They could re-evaluate Dad's consciousness once the medications had worked their way out of his system. The doctors didn't listen. They were in a rush to get him out of the CDU.

The course of Dad's treatment was based solely on conjecture and assumptions. There was absolutely no evidence to support what the doctors were about to do to him. His previous medical records weren't available, and no one had contacted his cancer doctor.

> **Bioethical Dilemma**
> - Impaired consciousness is one of the medical criteria that bioethics uses to determine whether or not an individual has quality of life.
> - By altering a person's consciousness with controlled substances and other lethal drugs, the practitioner is masking the true nature of that person's consciousness.

Maddie was told by Doctor Newman that Dad was end-stage and that the cancer had metastasized throughout his body. Maddie was beside herself with grief. She couldn't believe what the doctor was telling her. Only four days earlier, he was in remission.

Paula, on the other hand, was told something different. Doctor Robert had come into Dad's room and told her, "Your father's dying."

Paula said, 'Outside," motioning to the hallway. "We don't speak like that in here."

Paula followed the doctor to the end of the hall. Doctor Robert explained to her "Your father's cancer is in a bad place. It's very vascular." She told Paula that her father was going to bleed out and that it was time to call his family.

Paula cried. She remembered when her mother had been dying and wanted to make sure everyone had time to get there. She was in shock

Doctor Robert said, "We need to think about palliative care or hospice."

Paula told Doctor Robert, "My sister Maddie has Dad's power of attorney. She makes all the medical decisions." She indicated that Maddie wasn't at the hospital but that she would be back at three and the doctor could talk to her then.

Paula thought she was clear with Doctor Robert, but the doctor hadn't heard her. Her decision was already made. This was an eighty-year-old cancer patient with aggressive cancer and three admissions in two months. Doctor Robert went to the nurses' station and signed the order to send Dad to palliative care. Once the order was written, it became law; and nothing could restore Dad's inalienable right to "life, liberty and the pursuit of happiness"—not even Maddie or the *Declaration of Independence.*

> *The Declaration of Independence*
> July 4, 1776
>
> "We hold these truths to be self-evident, that all men are created equal, that they are endowed by their Creator with certain unalienable Rights, that among these are Life, Liberty and the pursuit of Happiness...."

16

"Death Warrant"

Maddie returned to the hospital about two P.M. Doctor Robert made no attempt to talk with her. Dad's death warrant had already been issued, and now it was only a matter of time before it would be executed.

Paula explained to Lynn and Maddie what had happened. They were both upset. Something had to be done. Meanwhile, a nurse came to discuss transferring Dad to the palliative care unit. She explained that their father needed special attention.

- Palliative care focuses on easing the patient's pain using pain management techniques and pain medications.
- Comfort care focuses on ensuring quality of life and physical as well as emotional and spiritual comfort for the patient.
- Hospice care for the terminally ill patient provides comfort measures as opposed to curative treatments. Hospice care can be provided in-home or in a hospice facility or a nursing home. Curative treatment protocols are no longer actively pursued, with the emphasis being on the administration of pain medications and comfort care.

Lynn and Maddie weren't aware of the implications of palliative care. Paula was insistent that her father wasn't ready for palliative care. She was furious that Doctor Robert had written the order without consulting Maddie. Paula felt the order was premature. She and Maddie both insisted that Dad was not end-stage and that only four days ago he was stage-three. It was as if nothing they said made any difference. All the hospital saw was an empty bed and someone to fill it.

The nurse told Paula, "I feel your pain."

Paula was indignant. "No, you don't. My father isn't dying."

The nurse gave Maddie her card, saying "You can call me at any time." She told them she could give them a tour of the palliative care unit if they wanted to see what it was like. Lynn and Maddie were upset with Paula. She wouldn't even consider the idea of palliative care.

After their meeting, Maddie requested a meeting with Doctor Newman to address some of their concerns. They met with Doctor Newman in the family room. Again Maddie and Paula insisted that Dad was not end-stage.

Doctor Newman explained, "The palliative care unit is a place where cancer patients with other medical conditions, like kidney or heart disease, go to be treated." He misled them into believing that palliative care was something that is wasn't.

Paula confronted Doctor Newman. "It's where you send people to die." Paula insisted that her father wasn't ready for palliative care. She asked the doctor, "Would you send a stage-two cancer patient to palliative care?" The doctor didn't answer her.

Again, Paula and Maddie tried to explain to Doctor Newman that their father was not end-stage. Maddie told him, "On Thursday, Dad was in remission, and now suddenly the cancer has spread all throughout his body." That didn't make sense to her.

Paula said, "You said all his test results came back negative." There was absolutely no evidence to support his end-stage diagnosis.

Doctor Newman continued to insist that their father was dying. Paula told him, "Everyone in this room is dying. It's not about dying. It's about healing. You're a healer and this is a healing facility."

The doctor was frustrated. "We can't keep your father here," he told them.

"He's a cancer patient," Paula responded. "Send him to the cancer floor."

The course of action was already decided. Doctor Newman couldn't change what Doctor Robert had done. He could only hear what he believed was Paula's denial and bargaining.

Paula felt boxed-in. Her father wasn't end-stage, and he wasn't ready for palliative care. She of all people would have compassion for him when it was time, but it wasn't time yet. She knew it. "You are not sending my father to a cancer ward," Paula exclaimed in desperation. Lynn and Maddie tried to reason with her. Paula wouldn't listen.

Maddie tried to take another approach with Doctor Newman. She asked, "Why wasn't Doctor Gita called?" Doctor Newman sat in silence.

Maddie continued, "I have faith in Doctor Gita. She has never lied to us." Maddie explained that if Doctor Gita told her that her father was end-stage and dying she would believe her, but she wouldn't believe anyone else.

Maddie demanded a consultation with Doctor Gita. "Isn't it amazing that no one bothered to call his cancer doctor?" she said. "He's a cancer patient."

By the conclusion of their consultation, Doctor Newman had agreed to a plan of action:

- Doctor Newman would consult with Doctor Gita. If Doctor Gita said their father was end-stage and dying, the family would believe her and act accordingly.

- The family would consider palliative care based on what Doctor Gita said.

- The family would meet with a hospice representative the next day to discuss how hospice might be able to assist them in taking care of their father. They were not informed that in addition to palliative care or hospice they had a third option, a home health care aide.

- The family wanted it entered into the chart that no one was to tell their father that he was dying.

Doctor Newman agreed with their plan. He indicated that he would ask for a consultation with Doctor Gita before any further action was taken regarding palliative care.

After their meeting with Doctor Newman, Lynn and Maddie insisted that Paula come with them to look at the palliative care unit. Paula was still very resistant, but she went reluctantly. When they got to the unit they learned that a room had already been reserved in their father's name even though they hadn't made the decision to have him transferred there.

The palliative care unit was an intensive care unit that had been remodeled for its current purpose. There were eight beds for terminally ill patients, such as cancer or AIDS patients. It was a place to die. All three of them reviewed a palliative care brochure and realized that they had been misinformed. Lynn and Maddie were very upset. They left with their minds made up. There was no way that Dad was going to this place.

That evening after Lynn left, Maddie and Paula took a break. They left Dad with Maddie's husband. They were only gone about ten to fifteen minutes. When they returned, they were surprised to find a gurney outside Dad's room. Maddie asked her husband if Dad had gotten a roommate.

Her husband told her, "No, they're here to take Dad to palliative care."

Maddie and Paula were outraged. Paula went to the nurses' station and demanded to talk to the nurse in charge. Paula explained to the charge nurse, Mercie that they hadn't agreed to send their father to palliative care. "You call

Doctor Newman right now," she told her. "Get him out of bed and tell him to come and spend the night in palliative care, so he can learn something about compassion."

Mercie heard Paula's anger and knew she was right. She followed Paula to Dad's room. Maddie was in the hallway with the paramedics. She was fuming. She told them in no uncertain words that they were not to transport her father. "You'll have to take him over my dead body," she informed them. "If you move him, I will call the TV news station."

The paramedics responded in unison, "We can't take him without your consent."

"You don't have my consent," Maddie responded.

Paula agreed with Maddie, telling Mercie, "What these doctors have done is not only immoral and illegal, but it's unethical." The paramedics left.

Maddie insisted that the hospital find a more suitable place for Dad. "He's a cancer patient; put him on the cancer floor or on the heart floor since he has heart problems."

Maddie looked straight at Mercie and told her, "Or if you have to, put him in a closet, but he is not going to palliative care. I wouldn't send my dying dog there if I had one."

Mercie assured them that their father would not be transferred to palliative care. "You can go home. They won't be taking him anywhere except to the heart floor," she promised them.

Dad was moved to the heart floor during the night. The following day more tests were done, but the results were all negative. Dad was still complaining about his stomach. Doctor Gita hadn't been called. It was a waiting game.

Meanwhile, Dad's mental state began to improve and he became more alert. He begged Maddie, "Don't let them give me any more pain pills. They gave me too much medicine. It made me hallucinate."

Dad continued to improve. His blood pressure stabilized. His creatinine decreased, and his infection cleared up. Maddie insisted everyone be upbeat. Dad's room was full of balloons, flowers and inspirational music. Lynn bought him an Uncle Sam doll to cheer him up and a purple hippopotamus. Maddie bought him sugar-free candy and balloons. Kiley and Sara came to visit Great Grandpa and played with his balloons. Sara sat on his bed and commandeered his hippopotamus. By the end of the visit, it was hers.

Kelly had come back as soon as she was told Grandpa was dying. She stood at Grandpa's bed and brushed his hair even though he didn't have any. He had always liked his hair brushed and when she was little, he used to pay her a quarter to brush it. Kelly did it now for free. Kelly was good with Grandpa. She used her wit and charm and feistiness to keep his spirits up. Grandpa liked a good fight, and Kelly and Maddie knew how to give him one.

Maddie turned up Dad's music and Paula closed the door. One of the nurses asked, "What's going on in that room?" Paula just smiled. The words of "Who Am I" reverberated throughout the room. Paula lay on the bed next to Dad's and tried to rest. She cried as Dad's favorite song played. She knew Who He Was. He was a humble man who wanted to live. Why couldn't she get Doctor Robert or Doctor Newman to see that?

When it was time to leave that night, Maddie's husband said he would stay so everyone could go home. Kirk was always considerate. He wanted them to go home and get some sleep.

The next day Maddie, Paula and Kelly met with the hospital's social worker and then with the hospice representative about Dad's discharge plans. Doctor Gita still hadn't been in to see Dad.

The hospice representative sold everyone on the fact that hospice could help. She explained their services and said that once Dad got better, they would leave. She offered hope, saying they had some patients in hospice for six months. One was in and out of hospice for four years. "We can assist you in taking care of your father," the representative told them. "And if he gets really bad and is about to die, we can arrange for a nursing home." Nothing was ever said about Medicaid and all the paperwork.

The hospice representative was very positive. She indicated that Dad would have twenty-four-hour nursing care, but she didn't explain that they were there to medicate him with lethal drugs. If Maddie had known, she never would have allowed them in her home. The hospice representative said they were there to keep their father "comfortable." Maddie didn't know that comfortable meant comfort care—which would end up being nothing less than euthanasia.

Maddie and Paula believed they were taking Dad home to get stronger so they could start radiation again in a couple of weeks. Doctor Gerald had told them that if they needed a couple weeks off, it would be okay. This was a family in crisis, and they needed help. By no means had they given up. They had given in only to the need for help.

Doctor Gita was on vacation. On the morning of Dad's release, Doctor Milton from her office came to see Dad. Doctor Milton examined him and concurred that a hospice evaluation was in order, and radiation should be stopped at that time. No one informed Maddie or Paula about his visit or his observations. Maddie was simply told that Doctor Gita's office was pulling out.

Doctor Milton didn't have access to Dad's records. He knew only what Doctor Newman told him. He was convinced to concur with a misdiagnosis. Dad was not end-stage terminal. He was very much stage-three in remission.

Later, when Doctor Gita returned from vacation and learned what they had done to Dad, she was outraged with shock and grief. She wanted to know, "What happened? He was doing so good? What doctor did this to him?"

17

Euthanasia

On July 9, Maddie brought Dad's walker to the hospital because he kept insisting he wanted to go for a walk. The nurses walked behind him. They couldn't believe he could walk so far. He kept walking and walking and walking. When he returned to his room, everyone stopped and clapped for him. It was a standing ovation for a very determined man.

Dad was having a hard time urinating, and Maddie told him that they would have to put the catheter back in if he couldn't go. He strained and tried hard, but he couldn't go. Dad asked for pain medicine to relieve the pain. The nurse told him that the pain was from the pressure on his bladder and medicine wouldn't help. They gave it to him anyway. The catheter was reinserted, and Dad's bladder was emptied. He passed a large amount of urine. Once the pressure was relieved, he felt better.

Dad was supposed to be released that day. Paula stayed home, getting everything ready. At about four P.M. Maddie was told that she could drive him home, but then the hospital spokespersons changed their mind because he needed oxygen. Dad was taken home by ambulance.

Maddie left the hospital believing that the hospice nurses could help her do all the things that needed to be done to get Dad stronger. She signed the paperwork and consented to let them in her home. What she didn't know was that she was taking her father home to die, not because he was dying but because that was the protocol that had been set forth for him. Doctor Robert's palliative care order was a precursor of death.

Over the next seven days, a series of caregivers would come and go. There were several times when there were holes in the schedule and they were left without coverage. The biggest battle over the next week would be to get the hospice nurses to realize that Dad was not end-stage, and to get them to stop drugging him with morphine and Ativan.

Dad got home about five o'clock. Everyone was waiting for him. He was tired and went to bed. The hospice nurse got there at seven.

Dad's first night home was very difficult. He hadn't eaten all day long. His blood sugar dropped to forty-seven, and the nurse kept shoving honey into his mouth to keep him from going into diabetic shock. Maddie checked his blood sugar every hour during the night. She wasn't sure whether or not to call 911, but Dad had said he didn't want to go back to the hospital.

"In and out! In and out!" he said about going back and forth to the hospital. He was tired of being poked and prodded. He just wanted to be home with his family with no more tubes or monitors and endless tests and doctors' orders.

After they got Dad's blood sugar under control, he began to improve. The next morning he actually got up and came to the table for breakfast.

Maddie told the hospice nurses, "Don't give him any pain medicine unless he asks for it, or I tell you to."

The hospice nurses kept using scare tactics like saying, "Your father is going to bleed out, but there won't be any pain" to justify giving him morphine and Ativan every three hours.

The following day, Dad got up and Maddie gave him a shower. He had enough strength to get into the shower with help. Maddie put lotion and powder on him, and he said he felt better.

Later, Maddie went out to run an errand for a neighbor. While she was gone, Dad went to the back porch and ate some ice cream. Dad was feeling better. He didn't want the oxygen anymore. While he was on the back porch, he pulled the oxygen tube out and refused to put it back in. Lynn came rushing inside. She said to Paula, "Dad took out his oxygen, and Kelly can't get him to put it back in." Paula went outside to help. Dad wouldn't listen to her either.

The next day, Patrick and Julie came over. Patrick spent some time with Grandpa. Grandpa had helped raise him, and Patrick was the apple of his eye. Dad saw in Patrick all the years of happiness that he had brought him and his wife, Viola.

Next, Julie went into Grandpa's room. She told him, "Don't worry, Grandpa, I'll take care of Kiley and Sara and Patrick; and I'll love them like you do."

Dad loved Julie for the strength and love she gave to his grandson and great granddaughters. He knew that she would honor her promise to him, and it made him happy.

After Patrick and Julie left, Paula insisted that Maddie and her husband go out to eat. Maddie needed a break. Paula told her, "I can get along without you for a couple of hours."

Maddie went reluctantly. While she was gone, Dad began projectile vomiting. The nurse tried to give Dad his nausea and secretion medicines, but he didn't want them. He tried to bite her. He thought she was trying to drug him again like when he was in the hospital. Paula asked her to try a rectal suppository. The nurse phoned the hospice office, and they called the pharmacy and ordered a rectal suppository. Lynn picked it up. It worked. Dad's nausea stopped.

Paula called Maddie and explained what was going on. She told Maddie to finish her dinner, but Maddie rushed home. "I shouldn't have left," Maddie said. Maddie didn't want to be away from Dad. She wanted to be with him all the time to make sure nothing happened to him.

Maddie kept insisting that the hospice nurses stop giving Dad morphine. She told the nurses that she thought he had a blocked bowel. "We need to get him cleaned out," she told them.

The nurses tried suppositories. Kelly heard Grandpa crying out, "Stop, you're hurting me." She ran into Grandpa's room and told them, "Cut it out! Don't hurt my grandpa." Kelly was Grandpa's protector.

The next day Maddie gave Dad an Ex-Lax because nothing the nurses were doing was working. They had given him Senakot, Docusate and Dulcolax, but nothing worked. The Ex-Lax didn't work either. Dad was still complaining of abdominal pain. The hospice nurse finally gave him some Dolomite.

Maddie told Dad, "I'm going to tell you the truth, that if you don't go to the bathroom, you will have to go back to the hospital or you are going to die."

After Maddie left the room, the nurse said, "He's going."

Dad immediately began having a large, gushing bowel movement. He discharged three inch-size rocklike masses that had been blocking his bowel. Once the blockage was relieved, Dad began to feel better. He was able to get out of bed and walk by himself. He appeared to be in good spirits.

On Thursday morning, the hospice doctor came. He took Dad's vital signs, which were normal, and said that because his vital signs were good the hospice staff was pulling out. Maddie asked the doctor to examine Dad's finger, which appeared to be broken. The doctor said it was probably gout from the chemotherapy. Maddie insisted it wasn't. Gout doesn't happen in two hours.

Later that day, Maddie told Dad she would take him shopping. Dad was excited. Lynn and Kelly stayed with Dad while Maddie and Paula left to run a few errands. While they were out, Lynn called Maddie on her cell phone. "The nurse just double-dosed Dad," she explained. Lynn was frantic.

"I said no medicine," Maddie told Lynn. Maddie hurried home.

When she got there, Dad had taken a turn for the worse. The nurse had double-dosed him with morphine and Ativan. Maddie confronted her, "Did you ask
him if he was in pain?"

"No," the nurse responded.

"Did he tell you he was in pain?" Maddie asked.

Again the nurse said, "No."

"Why would you give him a double dose?" Maddie asked angrily.

"Because he had a crease in his forehead," the nurse responded. "That's a sign
of pain. A sleeping patient is a comfortable patient," she added.

"His forehead is always creased," Maddie told her. "If he was in pain, he
would have asked for medicine."

Paula was upset too. "I have a creased forehead. I don't need morphine," she
told the nurse.

After the double dose, Dad went downhill quickly. He went into a kind of
semi-coma and slept all the time. He was on morphine and three other medicines
that caused drowsiness. He was dehydrated and nauseated. He didn't want to eat
or drink. The morphine was taking its toll on him. He was given enough morphine in seven days for seven and a half weeks. Morphine causes constipation,
nausea, vomiting, decreased appetite, decreased urine, apnea, cardiac and respiratory arrest. It should not be given with medications like Ativan.

Maddie was frustrated with the entire situation. "Fix him!" she demanded.
Maddie was beside herself. She insisted that the hospice nurses were trying to kill
Dad. Paula tried to calm her down.

After a visit with Dad, Maddie left his room in utter despair. She went to the
back porch and prayed. She asked God that if Dad were going to die to let her
know when. She picked up a Bible and randomly opened it to the story of "Paul's
last visit to Troas" (Acts 20:7-12).

It was the story of a young man who fell from a window while Paul was speak-
ing. Paul spoke until midnight on Saturday because he was leaving Sunday. The
young man fell from the third story, and everyone thought he was dead. Paul
went down and threw himself on the young man and told the onlookers not to
worry, that he was still alive!

Maddie was sad. She took it to mean Dad would die on Sunday. She shared
the verse with Paula. Paula focused on the part that he was still alive.

"Let's just enjoy him now," she said to Maddie. "He's still alive!"

On Saturday, Maddie went into Dad's room to look in on him. Dad looked
up and smiled at her and said, "Today's my birthday."

Paula saw Maddie in Dad's room with his singing teddy bear and his three happy birthday dolls and decided to join her. Maddie was next to Dad, and he was grinning from ear to ear. She played the happy birthday dolls, and everyone sang "Happy Birthday."

Next, Maddie's husband Kirk came in with the camera. He took pictures of this very special moment. Afterwards, Maddie lay next to Dad to comfort him. He sat up for a minute and rubbed her back. He was comforting her. Paula started to cry and had to leave the room. The odds of a miracle seemed to be diminishing.

Later, when they developed the film, a strange, bright light surrounded the head of Dad's bed. It was in every picture. Dad's bald head glowed with a yellow halo, and he looked angelic surrounded by Maddie and Paula and the light.

18

Into the Light

By Saturday afternoon, Dad's conditioned worsened and Paula called the hospice office. They sent an evening and a night nurse, but there was no one to cover Sunday morning.

At eight-twenty A.M., when Paula went in to check on Dad, he had a very noticeable death rattle. She knew what that meant. Dad needed to be suctioned. Paula called the hospice office and insisted that they send someone. "I have a delicate situation here," she told them. "I've got some very upset people. I need help."

"We don't have anyone" was their response.

Paula explained that her father needed to be suctioned. The hospice office sent a visiting nurse. The nurse examined Dad and ordered a suction machine. She had other patients to see and left. The machine was delivered to the house, but no one knew how to use it. Everyone was frantic.

Maddie, Lynn and Paula were nervous wrecks. It was hard to watch their father dying. Earlier, the hospice staff had given them a list of the signs of dying. Lynn memorized them and kept looking for every one. Paula told her to stop it, but once Paula heard the death rattle she knew it wouldn't be long. The morphine was taking its toll.

At one point, Maddie went into Dad's room. She looked out his window and saw the crows hanging around. She shooed them away. "Get out of here. You can't have him yet!" she scolded them. The birds left.

Complications of Morphine
•Constipation
•Nausea and vomiting
•Decreased appetite
•Decreased urine output
•Apnea
•Cardiac and respiratory arrest

About four P.M., the hospice nurse arrived. Annie was a gentle woman with a kind heart. She was a "death guide." She was there to provide support and comfort during Dad's final hours. Annie explained at every step what to expect. "Your father is on his path to God," she told them.

When Dad began to experience apnea, Annie prepared them for what would happen next. "Your father will stop breathing," Annie told them. "It will seem like he's gone, but he's not."

Annie was right. Dad stopped breathing four or five times. He rolled his shoulders as if trying to take off a tight garment. It was a gentle and an easy death. Suddenly Dad's eyes opened wide, and he looked up as if he saw someone above him. He wasn't blind anymore. He could see the room around him filled with his family and the light of God.

At the very moment when he took his last breath, his daughters were comforting him and releasing him to God. Maddie told Dad, "You're a winner. You've won what we're all here to claim. You've won your place in Heaven."

Paula explained to him what she had seen when she was dying. "God is going to enter the room. He's a being of light. When he asks you what you have done with your life, you will have many gifts to give him."

As Paula told Dad that God was a being of light, the entire room filled with a golden light. Paula said to everyone, "Look at the light."

All of the people in the room saw it. It entered the room at the exact moment that Dad took his last breath; and then as he exhaled and passed into eternity, it was gone. Annie said, "He's gone."

At six-forty P.M. on July 18, 2004, Paul Joseph Vertucci, Sr. died surrounded by his family. He didn't die from his cancer. He was murdered. By overdosing him with lethal drugs against his will, and against the will of his family, he was involuntarily euthanized.

His death certificate said he died of terminal stage esophageal cancer, but that wasn't true. He wasn't end-stage. He was stage-three in remission. It said he died of natural causes. They weren't. He was murdered because Florida law sanctioned it: It gives the medical system free rein to kill!

19

The Heart of the Matter

Dad died on Sunday. He wasn't in church, but church was all around him. He didn't die in a hospital hooked up to tubes and monitors. He died in the arms of his family surrounded by the people who were most important to him. He didn't die alone in a sterile environment. He died in a room full of laughter and tears, sorrow and joy.

He died in his own bed in the presence of his three daughters—Maddie, Lynn and Paula—his son-in-law Kirk who was like a son to him, and his grandson Patrick. When he died, everyone in the room saw the light of God. They not only saw it, but they were immersed in it.

Paula hadn't gotten her miracle, but she had witnessed a mystery. Embraced by the grace of God, she knew it was His own special way of letting them know Dad was still alive! The medical people could steal his body, but they couldn't take his soul. He was alive and well, dining at Jesus' table.

Lynn asked Annie if she had ever seen anything like this before. Annie answered, "I have seen many things but not this."

Dad's funeral was exquisite. Paula made a huge picture board of his life. It showed his wife Viola and pictures of his wartime service. There were pictures of his life in Ohio, but most of the pictures were of his life in Florida. There were pictures of him gambling in Las Vegas and Biloxi. He and Maddie took their annual gambling vacation. He was seen having fun at the ocean and dressed in a suit on a cruise with his family. He was captured fishing, golfing and celebrating birthdays. He was pictured at Kiley's and Sara's ballet recitals and playing with them on the back porch with water pistols and airplanes. He had a very good life with Maddie and Kirk. Maddie made sure Dad enjoyed his golden years. His joy and happiness were expressed in the pictures of his life.

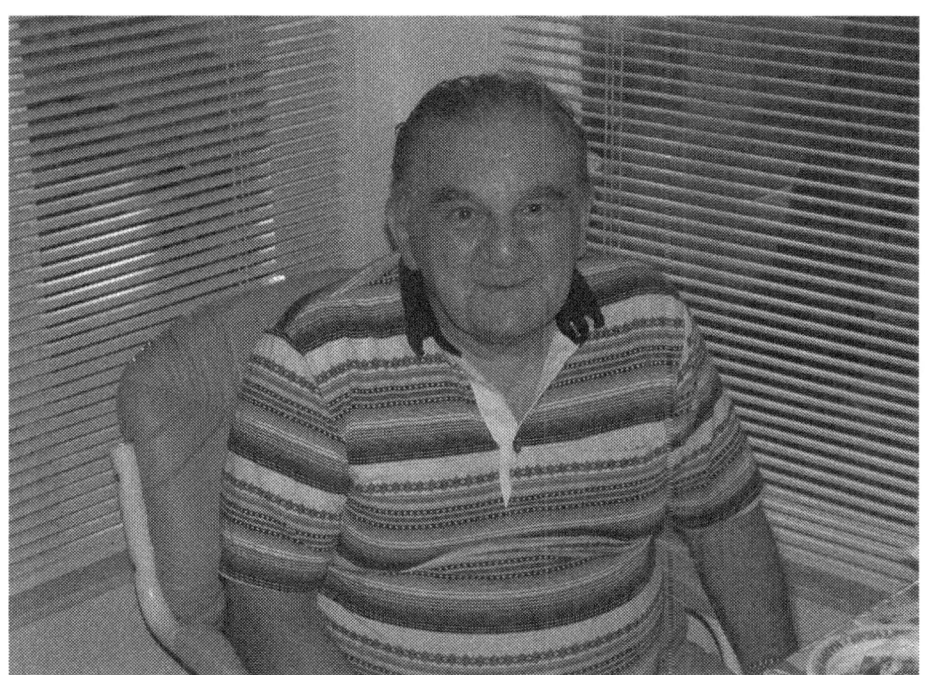

Dad didn't have a church service, and the priest wasn't available for his eulogy; but his funeral was unforgettable. People came with gifts that he had bought them and shared their memories with his family. People from the CITE center came to pay their respects. Kirk's family flew in from Washington, D.C., and Ohio. Allan and his family flew in from Ohio. Kelly was there with her two brothers. People from the bowling alley came. Postal workers from the Pine Castle Branch were there with friends and neighbors to offer their condolences and share their sorrow.

Maddie brought Dad's medal display case with his Bronze Star, and the bronzed last supper that he had made for her while he was at the blind school. His sisters and brothers bought him a rosary made of red roses for his casket. There were balloons to release to Heaven after the ceremony. Maddie and Allan were diligent about every detail of the celebration.

It was a dignified and loving service. After the minister spoke, people got up and shared their memories of this man called Pauley. They spoke of the wonderful gifts he had given them, and how his life had touched theirs. He helped pay for a court battle that meant a father would have custody of his daughter. He taught a boy how to fish and how to honor nature by throwing back the fish. This boy called him "grandpa" because Dad was the only grandpa he had known.

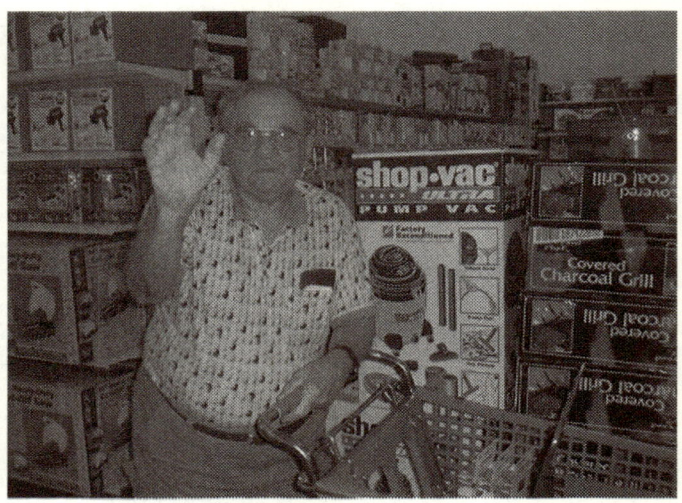

Lynn shared. His grandson Patrick told about Grandpa's generosity and love of shopping. Everyone laughed at stories of Dad's excessive buying. Paula spoke about who Dad was and how he was ushered into the light. When Dad's song "Who Am I" was played, everyone was touched. That day everyone knew a little more about who Dad was and what he had done with his life. His philosophy of life was clear, "Be good to people and be kind."

Even in death, he was still giving. As a tribute, his family passed out Bibles. The leftovers were taken to Doctor Gita's office where they were given to the staff and put out for the patients.

As they were leaving the funeral home after the service, Maddie remembered what Dad had said about church, and she knew he was in Heaven this very day with God and Mom.

Maddie and Dad were driving out of their neighborhood one Sunday on their way to go shopping. The trees were green and vibrant with life, and the grass was perfectly maintained and shimmering. The sky was blue and the warmth of the sun radiated down and covered the beautiful earth with its light.

Maddie asked Dad, "Dad, do you want to go to church?"

Dad answered, "No, I'm in church. This is church. I'm in God's church. You don't have to go to a brick building that man made. See the trees. See the grass. See the sky. This is God's church. It's in your heart. It's all around you."

"Got ya," Maddie replied.

Dad was right. Church is in the heart.

Church isn't in a building and Heaven isn't in the sky. Church is in the heart, and Heaven starts there too. Heaven is kept alive in the hearts and minds of God's people. Maddie and Kirk, Patrick, Julie, Kiley and Sara, Paula, Lynn, Joe, Allan and Kelly could all be at peace knowing that in that place their father, grandpa, and great grandpa dwelt.

Into the Light

By Paula Andrasko

In Memory of
Paul Joseph Vertucci, Sr.

You cannot fix everything by trying.
You cannot stop the rain or capture the wind.
You can try all you want, but time stops for no one.
You cannot fix everything by doing.
You cannot rewind time, or add another day to life
                                        by striving.
            You can try, and do, all you want,
                    but death comes for everyone:
Nothing can stop it from claiming what is its.
        Be still. Be silent. Look into the light
knowing that He who is the Author of your life
                    is also the Great Finisher.
Cry. Cry. Cry.

Death is stronger than man.
Death has taken him away from you.
It has robbed you of your time with him.
It is done.   The struggle is over.
He is gone and nothing you do, or try,
                            can undo death.
Grieve. Grieve. Grieve.

He is laid to rest. The battle is over.
Your hope has been dashed to death
                    by death itself and circumstance.
No more heroic attempts or drastic measures.

He has bridged the great divide.
Feel the pain of your loss, but do not suffer in its grip.
Feel. Feel. Feel.

Cry, grieve, feel.

Feel his presence everywhere.
In every rainbow, share his joy.
In every memory, touch his humanity.
In the warmth of his memory,
              let your spirit shine forth.
In the smile of a child express the true nature
                    of your love for him.
Share that love with someone who has no love
                that his love might live on.
   Do not blame God or the doctors or yourself.
Forgive. Forgive. Forgive.

No one was meant to be here forever.
Forever exists only in eternity.
Be still. Be silent. Dwell in that state of being
         where you and he are together again.
Drink in his being for whatever brief time
               you may have.
Share in his love. His compassion.
His kindness and generosity.
Share with the world his greatness.
Release. Release. Release.

Smile with the sacred knowledge
that he is not gone but that he lives.
He dwells among the clouds in castles in the sky
where eye has not seen and ear has not heard.
There in the center of God's loving hand,
he dwells in a place where kingdoms have no end,
             and death has lost its power.
              Honor him with your life.

Let go. Let go. Let go.

Forgive, release, let go.

Hold him forever in your heart.
He was your father, your son, your husband,
your grandfather, your neighbor and your friend.
He is all that he is, and all that he will ever be.
He has kissed the face of God and flies
        forever with His angels. He is free.
He has been resurrected with the wind.
          He soars with the eagles.
Be still. Be silent. Be happy for him.
Surrender. Surrender. Surrender.

In the quietness of today, spend some time with him.
Meet him in your dreams.
Know him in your heart of hearts.
You could not fix him by trying,
        or heal him by doing, or keep him
          with you by willing him to stay.
Release him. Release yourself. Release each other.
          Find peace again.
No one can die without God's permission.
Accept. Accept. Accept.

You are not separated in time and space anymore,
but only by "seeing" and "hearing" and then only
        for one last flicker of the candle
until he comes to usher you back home.
And in that moment, time will stop
and space will lose its hold on you.
You will shed this earthen vessel;
and put on a new and heavenly one
and drift away, up, up, up,
            toward the light,
        into the light,

                         away with the light
for all eternity dwelling in the light of the Lord
where He who gave you life awaited your return.
Heal. Heal. Heal.

Surrender, accept, heal.

PART IV
Recompense

It is the spirit of man and not the letter
of the law that keeps justice honest.
—Paula Andrasko

20

The Hippocratic Oath?

With the advent of bioethics and an agnostic approach to modern medicine, is the Hippocratic Oath still relevant? Did Doctor Robert and Doctor Newman solemnly swear to exercise their art solely for the cure of their patients, or has our drug-obsessed culture changed medicine from a healing profession into something else?

Are medical students still taught to practice their art with honor and uprightness, or is it not an art anymore, but just a business?

Can doctors still stay aloof and keep from wrongdoing and corruption, or can they be tempted by incentives and bonuses?

Are medical practitioners still here solely to help cure their patients, giving them no illegal drugs, or is it okay to legalize illegal drugs solely for comfort care and free enterprise?

Do doctors swear to honor their profession and reap prosperity and a good reputation by doing so, or is money more important than life and healing?

Are hospitals healing places anymore, or are they nothing more than big business with CEOs and insurance companies telling them what to do?

◆　　　◆　　　◆

When Paula was dying at the age of twenty-three, she went to her doctor. He had a copy of the Hippocratic Oath on his wall. She read it. It was charming and inspiring, but it took more than an oath or even her doctor to heal her. It took a miracle of God.

- **Paula believed in miracles.** Paula was a miracle. When the doctor told her she had a year to live, she didn't believe him and thirty-two years later by the grace of God she is still alive.

- **Lynn believed in miracles.** Lynn was a miracle. In the middle of the night, God reached in and took away her cancer.

- **Allan believed in miracles.** Allan was a miracle. After a near-fatal car accident that should have killed or crippled him, he is alive, sharing the Gospel with a hurting world.

- **Joe believed in miracles.** Joe was a miracle. After a bout with botulism in Nepal, he heard the angels singing and lived to tell about it.

- **Maddie believed in miracles.** Maddie was a miracle. On the operating table, when she was having surgery, she saw her body floating overhead and she knew she was gone; but God spared her and she lived to be her father's comforter in his hour of need.

They all believed in miracles. Dad was on his way to being a miracle. God wanted to perform one, but the bioethical machine of a managed health care system was more concerned about its bottom line. They killed him, and it was absolutely legal.

◆   ◆   ◆

My purpose is to heal my patient. I will do no wrong.

(Lynn) I know my father was not dying. We were going to go shopping that day. He was laughing and joking and then the hospice nurse double-dosed him, and he went into a drug-induced coma. They murdered him behind our backs. The insurance company didn't want to pay for him anymore. He was costing them a lot of money, and he was eighty and they thought he had lived long enough. They treated him no better than an animal that they would put to sleep. My father had the right to live. He paid his own insurance premiums, and he deserved to live his life to the fullest—no matter what his age. Who are these doctors that they can determine if a person should live and when a person should die? Are they doctors or are they God?

I will hold the profession of medicine sacred.

(Kelly) It was a lie. They totally misrepresented everything they said, including hospice. They said once they got him stronger, hospice would back out. It was like they were trying to help us, but they lied to us and murdered him.

I will practice my art solely for the good of my patient.

(Joe) It was malfeasance. It wasn't feasible for them to keep him alive. It cost them too much money to save his life. The insurance company wanted to protect their bottom line; and the doctors got their bonuses for not referring or treating him, so it was easier to murder him than heal him.

I will not give or peddle harmful drugs, no matter what.

(Maddie) They lied. We didn't think they were coming to our home to murder him. I can't believe they would come into our house, eat our food and murder our father in the next room.

I will honor my art in an upright manner.

(Paula) They took advantage of our feelings and our love for our father. We were emotional and upset. They didn't listen to us or hear what we were saying. The truth was that Dad was not end-stage. They were wrong. They ordered a man to hospice care because they were too busy and too greedy to seek the truth. It was criminal. They catered to the bottom line to collect their incentives and let an innocent man die before his time.

21

Disbelief

After Dad died and Doctor Gita learned about it, she called Maddie and left a message on her answering machine. "Maddie," she said, "I want to send my condolences. I just found out. We need to talk. Call me."

Maddie returned Doctor Gita's call, but Doctor Gita was with a patient. She tried again in several days.

On August 10 at eleven forty-five A.M., Maddie called and left a message. Doctor Gita returned her call in an hour.

"Madeline," Doctor Gita said, "I'm so sorry about Paul. I can't believe it. What happened? He was doing so good."

Maddie explained, "He was having trouble having a bowel movement and he passed out, so I called 911 and they took him to the hospital.

"Once the HMO doctors got hold of him they wanted me to just let him die from our first visit in April. At the hospital, they lied to us and told us he had end-stage cancer. They wanted to put him in palliative care. I said 'No.'" Maddie told Doctor Gita that she had wanted a consult with her, since she was treating Dad for his cancer. She had insisted that Doctor Gita needed to be involved with these decisions. "We requested numerous consults with you," Maddie said.

"No one ever called for a consult," Doctor Gita responded.

Maddie replied, "We kept telling the doctors that on July first Dad had his mid-point checkup with a CAT Scan, and we were told there was no spreading and the tumor had shrunk a little." Maddie explained that the cancer hadn't shrunk as much as they had hoped, but Doctor Gerald said that with the boost series of treatments the following week it should start shrinking.

"Dad was told it would be okay if he wanted a couple weeks off," Maddie added, "and he said, 'No. Let's keep going.' We were so excited that the cancer hadn't spread."

Maddie paused. "Doctor Gita, I want to ask you a question."

"What is that?" Doctor Gita asked.

"Did Dad have end-stage cancer?" Maddie inquired. "I need to know?"

Doctor Gita sounded shocked. "Absolutely not!" she exclaimed. "What doctor did this to him?"

"Doctor Ivan's office," Maddie responded.

"No," Doctor Gita said, "The doctor at the hospital?"

"Doctor Newman," Maddie told her.

Maddie made arrangements with Doctor Gita to pick up Dad's CAT Scan and medical records on Thursday.

Doctor Gita was outraged. She called the hospital and asked for Dad's physician. She spoke with Doctor Robert. When Doctor Gita asked the doctor, "What did you do to my patient?" Doctor Robert said, "I didn't do it. That was Doctor Newman."

Yes, Doctor Newman signed the death certificate, but Doctor Robert signed the order to place Dad in palliative care. It was Doctor Robert's order that started the death protocol that ended his life.

22

A Call for Justice

On August 12, almost a month after Dad's death, Maddie and Paula met with Doctor Gita at her office. Doctor Gita took them back into one of the examining rooms and hugged both of them. "I am so sorry," she said. "What happened?"

Maddie responded, "Dad had a bowel impaction. He was straining on the toilet and passed out for a few seconds. I called the paramedics. The last thing Dad said before going to the hospital was, 'Could someone give me an enema?'" Maddie explained that although the doctors had run tests, they hadn't done anything for Dad's constipation. They concentrated more on the cancer then the problem.

"They had his blood pressure meds out of whack, and he was overmedicated," Maddie continued. "Dad asked me to make them stop giving him the pain medicine. He said it was making him loopy and hallucinate."

Paula commented, "The doctors said Dad's consciousness was impaired. I told them to give him one more day. I asked them, what was one more day?" Paula indicated that she told Doctor Newman Dad was overmedicated. Dad's blood pressure had been running low, and he was on three blood pressure medications. "They put him on pain medicine," Paula added, "but he wasn't taking pain medicine at home."

Maddie informed Doctor Gita, "We requested the doctors contact you because you needed to be involved if they were sending Dad to palliative care." She explained that although she told Doctor Newman she would think about palliative care, she wanted Doctor Gita consulted to read the records and to confirm that Dad was end-stage.

"I didn't trust the HMO doctors," Maddie continued. "They are the ones that told me and my husband in April not to get any radiation or chemotherapy, that Dad had three to six months and just to let him go." Maddie indicated that she had been outraged at Jeanne from Doctor Ivan's office for telling her she was "inhumane" for trying radiation. "Doctor Ivan told us not to believe any doctor about radiation or chemotherapy," Maddie added, "because they don't work."

"I informed Doctor Newman," Maddie said, "that we would visit the palliative care unit, and if Doctor Gita agreed that Dad was end-stage, we would consider it. But if he went there, no one was to tell him he was dying. Doctor Newman agreed to consult with you before anything happened."

Doctor Gita responded, "No one called me."

"They said that you were backing out," Maddie told her.

Paula interjected, "Doctor Newman wrote in the records that he had consulted with Doctor Milton."

"Doctor Milton was not Dad's doctor, and he didn't know Dad's situation," Maddie asserted. "Doctor Milton just heard what Doctor Newman told him." Maddie told Doctor Gita that in the records, it had stated the family wanted all chemotherapy and radiation stopped, comfort only. "We said that until Dad was stable he couldn't have treatment," Maddie said, "that he could take two weeks off. We didn't know that comfort meant to overdose and murder him."

Maddie was indignant. "I feel since Doctor Ivan's office wanted Dad to die and be off the books, they helped to kill him."

Doctor Gita agreed. "They probably did. I will get you his medical records. What do you want?"

Maddie replied, "I want the CAT Scan from July first."

"I will get you any records you want," Doctor Gita assured her, "and I will help you in any way I can. I mean any way!"

Maddie responded that although her father was weak from radiation and chemotherapy and had problems eating, those were normal problems with his treatment.

Doctor Gita agreed with her, "Yes, he did have normal complications, but he was not end-stage."

Maddie asked, "The cancer didn't kill him?"

"No," Doctor Gita said, "The cancer didn't kill him."

"He would have had another good year, month, week or minute, but he was not end-stage," Maddie asserted.

Paula and Maddie thanked Doctor Gita for being so good to their father.

Doctor Gita summed it up, saying, "This should not have happened to Paul."

This would not have happened to Dad if Doctor Gita had been there. If she hadn't been on vacation, he would be in her office even now, spreading goodwill and making her laugh with another one of his practical jokes or making her smile with his kindness.

It took a law in Florida to end his life. The law protects the doctors and insurance companies and gives them free rein to make adverse decisions or medical mistakes without consequences when there is no spouse or a minor child under twenty-five years of age. Dad was excluded from protection under the Florida Wrongful Death Act because medicine is more powerful than justice.

23

Epilogue to Euthanasia

After the death of her father, Maddie Kisha began a search for legal help to file suit against the doctors who were involved with her father's treatment. Maddie and her brother Joe called more than twenty-five lawyers in two states, and they all said the same thing. Because she wasn't a spouse or a minor child under twenty-five years of age, she had no recourse to sue for malpractice or wrongful death. They all indicated she had an iron-clad case, but the Florida Wrongful Death Act excluded her from recompense.

Maddie and her brothers and sisters do not qualify under the law. Because they are over twenty-five, their claim has no validity. The fact that the law was established to limit damages for wrongful death has created a bottleneck of justice. When a patient is without survivors, according to the law, those involved in the victim's death are not required to pay legal consequences. As in the case of Paul Joseph Vertucci, Sr., this means that they can change a person's diagnosis and relegate them to a pain management or comfort care protocol that can end in death.

On the one hand, this is age discrimination. Is it fair that people over twenty-five do not have the right to seek recourse for actions that are not frivolous, but of a more serious nature, such as murder? Under the Florida Wrongful Death Act they cannot seek legal recourse. What started as a good thing has brought catastrophe. Secondly, the law has created a loophole that exonerates medical practitioners of liability and allows them to commit involuntary

---

Let Your Voice Be Heard!

- Wrongful Death is not frivolous.
- Taking away recourse for people twenty-five years old and older is age discrimination.
- Limiting liability and removing consequences, opens the door to euthanasia.

Involuntary euthanasia is murder!

euthanasia without consequences. Involuntary euthanasia is murder! By administering lethal and controlled substances against a person's will and against the will of their family, medical practitioners can violate our basic sense of decency and justice. The law has made it legal to commit sanctioned murder.

Because of the nature of managed health care in America, we are presented with a serious dilemma. Who is to be the judge of who should live and who should die? Should insurance conglomerates and powerful HMOs determine who is worthy and who is not? Should we allow doctors to put themselves in the place of God and write orders that deny a person his or her right to "life, liberty and the pursuit of happiness"?

By assigning our father to comfort care and hospice because the doctors deemed it advisable—and by misinforming his family about the true nature of these protocols—our father's inalienable rights were violated. By stating for the record that he was end-stage, he was denied treatment for treatable conditions: an impacted bowel and esophageal cancer. For although esophageal cancer in rarely curable, it is treatable.

After her father's death, Maddie and her brother Joe researched their father's cancer staging. He was a stage-three cancer patient, but his cancer was contained, and it had not spread throughout his body. He was in remission. There was no medical evidence to substantiate the doctor's misdiagnosis that he was end-stage. In fact, there was evidence in writing to substantiate that he was in remission and could look forward to up to five more years of life.

At the time the end-stage misdiagnosis was made, Dad's previous medical records were not accessible. The doctors in charge of his treatment failed to do due diligence and speak with his cancer specialist or procure his medical records. They relied on their own judgment to change his staging to end-stage. In the course of four days, he went from a stage-three cancer patient in remission to end-stage metastasized.

The doctors in charge neglected to treat him for his presenting condition, an impacted bowel, but rather chose to focus on the fact that he was eighty and a cancer patient with an incurable—but treatable—cancer, and that he had cost his HMO a considerable amount of money. He had been hospitalized three times in two months. He choked on a hot dog. He bled from his radiation. He had an impacted bowel. None of these caused his death. Anyone can choke. Anyone can bleed. Anyone can have an impacted bowel. These are not issues that would be considered end-stage.

However, the HMO doctors who managed Dad's case determined it prudent to send him home—without treating his impacted bowel—and condemned him to death through comfort care. Hospice is a valid movement, and many patients are end-stage and need comfort care, but that was not the case for Dad. Dad was overdosed with morphine and Ativan. Morphine is illegal and Ativan is a controlled substance. The hospice nurses continued to force these medications on him against the wishes of his family.

Maddie insisted that Dad didn't need pain medicine. He was given enough morphine to harm a healthy person. Morphine shuts down the kidneys. Dad had renal insufficiency. Morphine shuts down the respiratory system. Dad had fluid on one of his lungs. Morphine stops the heart. Dad had congestive heart failure. His conditions were all under control with medication. Morphine should have been contra-indicated in his case. His situation did not require pain management, except for the pain that was created by his impacted bowel.

If you went to the hospital for an impacted bowel, would you want the doctors to give you morphine for the pain? If your father had cancer, would you want the doctors to change his diagnosis and send him home to die? If your elderly mother had a serious illness, would you want the doctors to sign her death warrant because the insurance company demanded it?

We hope that by reading our father's story you have gained a better understanding of what could happen to you or someone close to you. Our hope is that you have grown to know our father as we did and to love him for the special person that he was. It is our desire that you imitate him and remember to "be good to people and be kind;" but moreover, our goal is to leave you with a few simple things to consider if you or someone close to you is diagnosed with cancer or another serious illness.

Do not take your symptoms lightly. If you experience the symptoms of acid reflux, have it assessed by a doctor whom you can trust. GERD (gastroesophageal reflux disease) if left untreated can result in serious complications like Barrett's disease. Barrett's disease is the growth of intestine cells into the esophagus and can lead to cancer of the esophagus. Esophageal cancer is rarely curable but it is treatable.

Do not be afraid to ask for a second option. Cancer is growing at epidemic rates in American today. If you or someone close to you is diagnosed with cancer, you need to know your options. Don't lose hope. Make sure you understand what stage you are in and what you can expect during your treatment. If you have a concern about your diagnosis or prognosis, ask your doctor for a consultation with another doctor to confirm their assessment of your case. It is your life, and you have an inalienable right to life. Don't take that right lightly, and don't let anyone else take that right lightly. Don't let insurance companies and HMOs deny you your right to live.

Do not be afraid to question your insurance company. If you are denied treatment under your insurance, do not be afraid to appeal the decision. Educate yourself about your insurance, and if feasible supplement your coverage with other coverage to protect you in the event of a catastrophic illness like cancer. Don't take no for an answer. If you need help in maneuvering the insurance maze, ask someone to be your advocate to help you get the care and treatment that you need and want.

Do not believe everything you are told. If you have a terminal illness and are told you only have so much time to live, first of all, don't fall prey to that kind of fatalistic thinking. No one can tell you how much time you have. The doctors are only making educated guesses, but they are just that—guesses. The only one who knows how much time you have is God. Put your life in order, but don't give up simply because someone else told you that you are dying. Believe in miracles. Have hope! God is still a healing God, and people have survived the very illness or disease that you are dealing with. You are not a statistic; you are a person.

Make your wishes known. If you have a terminal illness, be prepared. Make your wishes known to those around you. Create a will. We are all finite. Every one of us will die at some time or another. Think about a living will and a do-not-resuscitate order, but do not ignore the need for an advance medical directive. An advance medical directive allows you to spell out under which circumstances you would want to be treated and under which you would rather not. A living will without an advance medical directive could mean that you will die under circumstances that you might not have chosen.

Find an advocate to help you through your illness. If you face a life threatening illness, find someone you trust to be your advocate. Let that person know what is going on with you and what you expect from your doctors. If you are designated as someone's medical advocate, be there for that person during the illness and treatments. If the person is hospitalized, be actively involved and visible. If the doctors make unwise or adverse decisions, stand up to them. Hospitals generally have an ombudsman who can facilitate maneuvering your way around the system should disagreements arise. Yell loudly and don't shut up. If you feel your rights are being violated, call 911 or the police. This is your life or the life of someone close to you.

Get involved and fight injustice wherever you find it. When a country falls asleep and becomes indifferent or indulgent, it can fall prey to people or circumstances that promote injustice. Stand up for what is right. Euthanasia is murder.

> **Take a Stand Against Injustice!**
>
> Visit http://www.hospicepatients.org/euth-center.html to find a sample letter protesting involuntary euthanasia.

Murder is illegal. Learn more about what you can do to stop the threat of euthanasia. Write your congressman, senator or the President. Start a petition to stop euthanasia. Keep current on this and other important issues, and let your voice be heard.

"Be good to people and be kind." Take time to be good to people. Practice random acts of kindness as often as you can. Every day is precious. Make sure you let the people you love know how you feel about them. Tell them you love them and express that love often. No one is guaranteed another day. Today might be your last day. Treasure each and every day and shower everyone you meet with love and kindness.

Acknowledgements

We would like to thank the many people who supported us and came to our assistance during Dad's battle with cancer. Special thanks to Kirk, who was with us throughout Dad's illness. Thanks for your consideration and sacrifice. You were with us at the hospital and in emergency. You helped us to make sure that Dad had everything he needed. You were like a son to him. You were his golfing buddy and his friend. You helped to make his years in Florida happy, and we thank you!

Added thanks to the following people who gave of their time and resources, love and understanding: Thomas Andrasko, Lynn Brown, Joe Vertucci, Allan Vertucci, Sr., Patrick, Julie Duffy, Kiley, Sara, Joseph G. Kisha, Aunt Madeline, Kelly Sturgill, Carol Kinelski, Karen Kelly, Suze Parker, Julie Vaccarella and Charlie Lambusta. Special thanks to Dad's friends, Ollie, Kristine and Dick. Without all of your kindness and compassion our battle would have been unbearable.

An additional thanks to Scott Caldwell for his support after our father's death.

We also want to thank the following groups: the Pine Castle Post Office for their support, prayers and numerous acts of kindness; the Veteran's Administration, the CITE center, and the School for the Blind in Birmingham, Alabama, and West Palm Beach, Florida, for the services and affectionate care they provided our father.

Special thanks to the members of the armed services. Thank you for protecting us and keeping the world free for democracy. To the survivors of the Holocaust, we hope that time has lessened the insufferable agony that you endured. And to Bob and Mary Schindler and their family, we offer our condolences on the loss of their beloved daughter Terri Schiavo. We are sorry! We wish you and the survivors of the Holocaust peace, joy and happiness!

And finally, to our beloved father, Paul Joseph Vertucci, Sr., we feel your presence everywhere. Thank you for all the things you did for us, but most of all for being who you are. We know that you would want us to share your story with the world. We love you! We miss you! Save a place for us at Jesus' table!

Doctors' Acknowledgement

A special thanks to Dr. Barry Jones who was both honest and supportive during Dad's illness. There are still many caring physicians, and we wish to thank them for their continuing efforts to heal and cure their patients. Doctor Jones loved Dad and heard his suffering. To doctors everywhere, we ask that you listen to your patients. They are sometimes the best authority on their conditions.

To the real Doctor Gita and Doctor Gerald, thank you for your compassion, for your love and for your commitment to your profession. To the others who assisted us with Dad's treatments and medical care, thank you for your dedication and hard work, especially the nurses in the chemotherapy room and the radiation technicians. To the doctors and medical practitioners whose names have been changed to protect their anonymity, we offer this book in hopes that next time you might do better. Never forget the sanctity of life, and always remember to offer dignity and respect to everyone who comes your way. We seek justice, but above all else we offer kindness.

About the Authors

Paula Andrasko came to Florida during her father's illness to help take care of him during his radiation and chemotherapy treatments. She spent the last nine weeks of her father's life caring for him and sharing her faith, hope and love. Paula is a writer and speaker in the area of death and dying. Since having a near death experience in 1972, Paula's mission has been to share God's love and light with as many people as possible. She is currently finishing her next book, *Near Death Revelation,* and has begun work on her third book, *God is Bigger than Bulimia.*

Maddie Kisha was her father's caregiver and advocate during his courageous battle with cancer. Maddie is a citizen's advocate and has promoted legislation in Florida to protect citizens from identity theft. She also worked with the Florida Consumer Action Network Foundation to educate citizens about new legislation and its effect on them.

Both Paula and Maddie believe that one person can make a difference. It takes only one person to take action in order to set the wheels of justice moving. One person affecting another person makes justice honest and kindness possible.

Both women have been active in their own communities in helping to bring about change through social action. Paula helped to bring about justice for a young boy who was shot to death simply because he was walking home and was in the way of a gang-related feud between two rival posse members. He was shot in the heart and died almost instantly. Paula went door-to-door to petition the Juvenile Court in Akron, Ohio to consider the minor perpetrator as an adult. Her action stirred public sentiment and helped to bring about justice.

Maddie helped to ensure that identity theft would be taken seriously in Florida. Her efforts supported the passage of legislation that ensures legal action against individuals who write bad checks or commit identity theft.

You can contact the authors at:

Maddie Kisha or Paula Andrasko
P.O. Box 592013
Orlando, FL 32859

APPENDIX

Bible
American Bible Society
http://www.bibles.com/

Audio-Bible
http://www.audio-bible.com/bible/bible.html/

Bioethics
Center for Practical Bioethics
http://www.midbio.org/

Nuffield Council on Bioethics
http://www.nuffieldbioethics.org/

Transplant-medicine ethics
http://www.nationalreview.com/smithw/smith200410200349.asp

Cancer-related issues
Association of Cancer Online Resources
http://www.acor.org/

Barrett's disease
http://pathology2.jhu.edu/

Esophageal cancer
http://www.cancer.org/

Gastroesophageal reflux disease (GERD)
http://www.webmd.com/

National Institute of Cancer
http://www.nci.nih.gov/

Catholic-related subjects
Encyclopedia of Religious Topics
http://www.newadvent.org/

Novenas, etc.
http://www.catholicdoors.com/

Consumer and patient protection websites
Agency for Healthcare Research and Quality
http://www.ahcpr.gov/

Center for Medical Consumers
http://www.medicalconsumers.
org/pages/PATIENTSAFETYSTILLANELUSIVEGOAL.html

Florida Consumer Action Network
http://www.fcan.org/

Floridians for Patient Protection
http://www.floridiansforpatientprotection.org/

Health care choices
http://healthcarechoices.com/rolfiling/profile fl.htm

Health care directives (forms)
http://www.hcdecisions.org/

Elder protection and resource websites
Topics for Seniors/Firstgov
http://www.firstgov.gov/Topics/Seniors.shtml

National Center on Elder Abuse
http://www.elderabusecenter.org

National Institute on Aging
http://www.nia.nih.gov/

Euthanasia and related medical issues
Assisted Suicide/United Press International
http://washingtontimes.com/upi-breaking/20041109-014543-1627r.htm

Assisted suicide/euthanasia
http://www.weeklystandard.com/Content/Public/Articles/000/000/0004/47lzche.asp

Drug reactions/CNN health
http://www.cnn.com/HEALTH/9804/14/drug.reaction/index.html

Euthanizing children/The Daily Standard
http://www.weeklystandard.com/Content/Public/Articles/000/000/004/616jszlg.asp

International Task Force on Euthanasia
http://www.internationaltaskforce.org/ascc/htm

Medical errors/CNN health
http://www.cnn.com/HEALTH/9911/29/medical.errors/

Medical mistakes/CNN health
http://archives.cnn.com/2000/HEALTH/04/28/thin.white/

Terri Schiavo case/St. Petersburg Times
http://www.sptimes.com/2004/11/02/Tampabay/Michael_Schiavo_tirin.shtml

Government websites
The United States House of Representatives
http://www.house.gov/

The United States Senate
http://www.senate.gov.

Holocaust
United States Holocaust Memorial Museum
http://www.ushmm.org/

Hospice
Hospice Patients Alliance
http://www.hospicepatients.org/

Veterans information
National veterans cemeteries
http://www.cem.va.gov/

Wartime service
The 89th Infantry Division
http://www.89infdivww2.org/

Index

A

Acid Reflux xiii, 97
Adenocarcinoma 20
Advance Medical Directive 98
Advocate 105
Agnostic xiv, 87
Andrasko, Paula xiii, xiv, 1, 13, 55, 80, 85, 105
Angel stone 39
   also see lucky charm
Ativan xiv, 69, 70, 71, 72, 97

B

Baby boomers xv, 17
Barrett's disease xiii, 19, 97, 107
Bible 72, 107
Bioethics xiv, 16, 87, 107
Bronze Star 16, 47, 77
Burial benefits 3

C

Cancer cross 34, 43
Casting Crowns 50
   also see Who Am I
CAT Scan 54, 90, 91, 93
Catastrophic illness 98
Chemotherapy xiii, 16, 20, 21, 22, 24, 27, 33, 36, 38, 42, 43, 47, 48, 49, 50, 53, 54, 92, 93, 103, 105
Comfort care xiii, xiv, 17, 67, 87, 95, 96, 97
Consciousness
   Impaired 19, 61, 92
   state of xv, 81
Constipation 52, 72, 92

Cost-containment 20, 22
Critical Decision Unit (CDU) 60

D

Death warrant xi, xii, 63, 97
Declaration of Independence
   Life, liberty and the pursuit of happiness 62, 96
   also see inalienable rights
Diabetic retinopathy 18
Do-not-resuscitate order 59, 98

E

Esophageal cancer 107
   also see end-stage
Esophagogastrectomy 21
Euthanasia
   involuntary xiv, 95, 96
   passive xiv

F

Feeding tube 21, 33
Florida National Cemetery 3
Florida Wrongful Death Act 95
   also see minor child
   also see spouse
Floridians for Patient Protection xiv, 108

G

Gastroenterologist 30, 34
GERD (gastroesophageal reflux disease) xiii, 97
Grief 68
   also see grieving

H

Health Maintenance Organization (HMO) xiii
Heimlich maneuver 29
Hippocratic Oath xiv, 87
Hitler 6, 15, 16, 44
Holocaust 109
    also see Auschwitz
    also see Terezan
Home health care aide xiii, 65
Hope 9, 16, 17, 18, 20, 22, 30, 31, 33, 34, 38, 43, 44, 46, 50, 51, 54, 67, 80, 97, 98, 101, 105
Hospice care xi, xiii, xiv, 17, 89

I

Impacted bowel xiii, 17, 59, 96, 97
Infant of Prague 36, 37

K

Kisha, Maddie xiii, xiv, 95, 105

L

Light of God 32, 42, 75, 76
Living will 59, 60, 98
Lortab 60
    also see Vicodin

M

Macular degeneration 18
Malpractice xiv, 95
Managed health care 96
Medical liability xiv
Miracle(s) 16, 22, 31, 43, 44, 46, 73, 76, 87, 88, 98
Monet, Claude 19
Morphine xiv, 60, 61, 69, 70, 71, 72, 74, 97

N

Near death experience 23, 105
Neupogen 54
Novena(s) 37, 38, 39, 45, 108

O

Ohrdruf 4, 15, 16, 26

P

Pain management xiii, 95, 97
Palliative care 93
    also see palliative care unit
Port 36, 48
Post traumatic stress 16
Power of attorney 59, 61
Prayer(s) 9, 23, 30, 44, 45, 50, 51, 101
    also see fleece
Procrit 50, 53, 54
Protocol xiii, 69, 91, 95

Q

Quality of life 20, 42

R

Radiation xi, xiii, 16, 17, 20, 21, 22, 24, 27, 33, 42, 43, 45, 47, 48, 49, 50, 53, 54, 67, 92, 93, 96, 103, 105
Random acts of kindness 49, 57, 99
Raphael 37
    also see archangel
Right to die xv
Right to live xv, 22, 88, 98

S

Sacraments
    communion 9, 46, 47
    last rites 47
Signs of dying 74
    also see death rattle
St. Therese of the Little Flower 44
Stent 33, 34, 36, 38, 39, 53

T

Truman, Harry S. 11

V

Vagus nerve 59

Vertucci, Paul Joseph vii, xi, xiii, xiv, 3, 6, 75, 95, 101
   also see Pauley

Veterans
   Administration 19, 101

Veterans of Foreign Wars (VFW) 4

Vietnam War 7, 15, 16

W

White light 42

World War II
   crossing the Rhine River 6, 47
   also see Camp Miles Standish

Wrongful death v, xiv, 94, 95

978-0-595-34041-5
0-595-34041-5